ENDORSEMENTS

"I found this book to be a fun, practical, easy-to-read guide on helping an applicant find their voice for their personal statement. Using a clear, systematic approach supported by examples, Dr. Gray unveils the true purpose of the personal statement and why it's so important for an applicant to know oneself. I think the process through which he guides the reader will prove beneficial not only for the personal statement but for the medical school interview as well. Perhaps even more valuable is that the reader will achieve a better understanding of one's motivations for pursuing a career in medicine."

Gregory M. Polites, MD
Associate Professor of Emergency Medicine
Chairman of the Central Subcommittee on Admissions
Washington University School of Medicine

"Another superb book from the Premed Playbook series by Dr. Gray. This edition helps medical school applicants approach the personal statement with confidence and inspiration. This is done through easy to read explanations of all relevant topics from beginning to the end. Furthermore, the different stages of drafts with edits are incorporated to elaborate what can seem as ambiguous feedback to applicants. A beginning pre-health advisor looking to get caught up with personal statements would benefit tremendously from reading this book!"

Joon Kim, EdD
Director of Postbaccalaureate Premedical Certificate Program
Keck Graduate Institute

"Dr. Gray is a wonderful source of guidance and reliable advice on the premed journey. Dr. Gray is a gift to premeds. He is a guide for what is often a long, arduous, and taxing journey."

Sujay Kansagra, MD
Author of *The Medical School Manual,*
Everything I Learned in Medical School,
and Why Medicine

The Premed Playbook
Guide to the Medical School Personal Statement

THE PREMED PLAYBOOK

GUIDE TO THE MEDICAL SCHOOL PERSONAL STATEMENT

Write Your Best Story. Secure Your Interview.

Ryan Gray, MD

NEW YORK

LONDON • NASHVILLE • MELBOURNE • VANCOUVER

The Premed Playbook Guide to the
Medical School Personal Statement

Write Your Best Story. Secure Your Interview.

Published in New York, New York, by Morgan James Publishing. Morgan James and The Entrepreneurial Publisher are trademarks of Morgan James, LLC.
www.MorganJamesPublishing.com

The Morgan James Speakers Group can bring authors to your live event. For more information or to book an event visit The Morgan James Speakers Group at www.TheMorganJamesSpeakersGroup.com.

ISBN 9781683508533 paperback
ISBN 9781683508540 eBook
Library of Congress Control Number: 2017960665

Cover Design by:
Rachel Lopez
www.r2cdesign.com

Interior Design by:
Paul Curtis

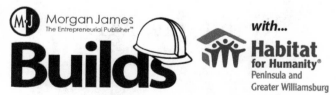

In an effort to support local communities, raise awareness and funds, Morgan James Publishing donates a percentage of all book sales for the life of each book to Habitat for Humanity Peninsula and Greater Williamsburg.

Get involved today! Visit
www.MorganJamesBuilds.com

To my daughter, Hannah,
who has me in awe every day.

DOWNLOAD MORE PERSONAL STATEMENTS

There are many more personal statements with my feedback that I couldn't include in this book that you can download 100% FREE at personalstatementbook.com/bonusessays.

TABLE OF CONTENTS

ACKNOWLEDGEMENTS

I want to thank the amazing community of premed students who helped with this book. My launch team, and others, came together and gave me direct feedback to help craft the message in this book to make it better for you. There were several students who went above and beyond with their dedication and feedback, including Chris Felici, Diane Ghanem, Evelyn Guerra, Hunter Graham, Kathrine Mansfield, Kelley Bellia, Magnus Chun, Michael Locascio, Miriam Moctezuma, Nguyen Nguyen, Regina Heit, Suzanne Chaar, Sylvia Okonofua, Tanya Panwala, Tia Gray, and William Haug.

INTRODUCTION

Why is it that we can write essays on world issues or book reports without any problems, but when it comes to writing about ourselves for our personal statement, we freeze up and stare at a blank screen forever?

You would think that writing about a topic that you have intimate knowledge of would be easy. But it's not. Or at least we don't make it easy for ourselves.

Where are you supposed to start? What are you supposed to write about? How are you supposed to cram 20, 30, 40 or maybe more years of your life into 5,300 characters, or even 4,500 characters? The answer to that last question is simple: you don't.

The personal statement is not supposed to be a timeline of your life. It's not meant to be an essay form of your résumé. The problem is that most students approach it like it is. They try to tell their entire story in such a small amount of space.

The result of that is a mess. Anyone who has lived longer than a decade can't possibly fit their journey into the format the American Medical College Application Service (AMCAS) and American Association of Colleges of

Osteopathic Medicine Application Service (AACOMAS) dictate. Those services allow you 5,300 and 4,500 characters, respectively. The Texas Medical and Dental School Application Service (TMDSAS) allocates 5,000 characters.

So many students I talk to see these character limits and just freeze. They hear other student's claims about telling *the story* of their lives and just can't fathom doing that in so few characters.

I'm here to tell you that you don't have to tell your life story. You don't have to create a beautiful story that has a beginning, middle, and end. Your personal statement is not a creative writing piece. It's a reflection on your journey and what you have learned about yourself.

It's a story about why you want to be a doctor. It's a story about the impact you want to make in your community. That is the story you have to tell. It is the *only* story you have to tell. That is all you need to get across to the Admissions Committee. If you aren't doing that, then you have failed.

I asked Dr. Rafael Rivera, Associate Dean for Admissions at NYU Langone Medical Center, about his thoughts on the personal statement. Here is what he had to say:

> *To be impactful, the personal statement needs to provide Admissions Committees with important insights into why an applicant has chosen to devote his/her life to medicine, and how they hope to improve the lives of those around them by means of their work as a physician.*

Why have you chosen to devote your life to medicine? What do you hope to accomplish as a physician? When you put it like that, it seems pretty straightforward, yet most students are failing to do this.

Writing your personal statement is hard. It takes a while. You need to take breaks from writing it, allow yourself space to reflect on it and return to it with fresh eyes. It requires you to know yourself, know your motivations, and know why you are embarking on this journey.

The personal statement is a very important part of your medical school application, and you shouldn't leave it until the last minute.

This book will show you how to start generating ideas for your personal statement. It will show you how to narrow down what you will want to write about. It will help you put it all together so that when the reader—the Admissions Committee member who controls your destiny—is done reading your personal statement, he or she will truly understand why you want to be a physician. This book will help you reflect on your journey, forcing you to look deep inside yourself to pull out the best ideas. It will show you real examples of personal statements that I have reviewed and commented on so you can understand where some students go right and others go wrong.

When you are done reading this book, you'll have everything necessary, from initial ideas to final draft, so that you can be confident submitting your personal statement with your medical school application.

YOUR EXPERIENCES AREN'T ENOUGH

Most early drafts of personal statements that I read are boring. The majority of them tell one of a few different stories. The first is the common story of personal or family illness that exposed the student to medicine either early in life for traditional students or later in life for nontraditional students. A second common story is the premed student who has always known that she is supposed to be a physician.

The fact that most personal statements are boring has nothing to do with the common journey students take to get to the point of applying to medical school. Don't let that dissuade you from having a personal statement that you think will sound like others.

If you look at most movies, they follow a common theme as well. The Hero's Journey is a common pattern found in storytelling created by Joseph Campbell. Popular movies and stories like *Star Wars*, *The Matrix*, and even *Harry Potter* all follow the progression of the Hero's Journey. Just because they follow this theme doesn't mean that they are boring and people don't want to watch or read these stories.

If the audience knows the standard template of a movie, why do they continue to watch these movies? It all has to do with the storytelling. If the writer does a great job of telling the story, they can draw the audience in by engaging their different senses.

With this book, I'm going to show you how to engage the reader with this type of great storytelling. Even if your journey to medicine is similar to another student's, you will learn how to _show_ the reader why and how your experiences have made an impact on you. You'll be able to engage the reader's different senses, causing your personal statement to be memorable. Follow what this book lays out, and you can ensure your personal statement won't be boring and will stand out from the rest.

STORYTELLING

SECTION I

THE KNOWLEDGE

CHAPTER 1

APPLICATION PROCESS OVERVIEW

The personal statement is part of the medical school application. I think it's important to provide a general overview of the application process before we dive into the specifics of the personal statement.

The medical school application process is very confusing for most students. The process includes primary applications, secondary applications, essays upon essays, interviews, and so much more. *This is by no means an exhaustive account of what is required. I highly recommend you listen to The Premed Years[1] for more detailed information.*

Timing

Traditional applicants apply to medical school the summer before, or at the start of, their senior year to start medical school almost immediately after they graduate from college. That means that if you are graduating from college in May of 2024, hoping to start medical school in August of 2024, you will be applying

[1] http://www.premedyears.com

to medical school starting in May and June of 2023. Yes, the application process is that long! The primary application is usually open from May/June to October.

The first thing to keep in mind is that while medical schools give you deadlines by which to submit your primary application, you should consider forcing yourself to apply within the first couple months of the application cycle opening. The majority of US medical schools interview, and admit, students on a rolling basis. This factor means that the sooner your primary and secondary applications are turned in and complete, the sooner your file is reviewed. Then, the sooner your file is reviewed, the sooner you'll, hopefully, be invited for an interview. And, of course, the sooner you are invited for an interview, the sooner your application will be discussed to determine if the Admissions Committee wants to accept you, put you on a waitlist, or reject you. Don't make the mistake of applying late. It is the most common, preventable mistake that students make in the application process.

MCAT

You should plan to take the MCAT no later than March or April of the year you are planning on applying. Doing so will allow you to get your score back before you submit your application. If you need to delay your test to make sure you are prepared, that is okay; just understand that the longer it takes for your MCAT score to be received by the medical school, the longer it will take for your application to be complete. You should still plan on submitting your application early, even if you're taking the MCAT later. Don't sacrifice your MCAT score just to take the MCAT earlier. A poor score on the MCAT will do you a lot more harm than a last-minute application. Read *The Premed Playbook: Guide to the MCAT* [2] for more information on the MCAT.

Different Application Services

There are three different US application services available, depending on which medical schools to which you will want to apply. Canada also has a very fragmented application service depending on the schools you want to apply to there.

---

[2] http://www.mcatbook.com

In the US, if you are applying to an allopathic (MD) medical school, you will use the American Medical College Application Service (AMCAS) for almost all of the MD granting schools.

If you are applying to osteopathic (DO) medical schools, you will use the American Association of Colleges of Osteopathic Medicine Application Service (AACOMAS) for almost all of the DO schools.

The exception to these application services is Texas medical schools.

Texas has the Texas Medical and Dental School Application Service (TMDSAS). The TMDSAS serves all public medical school in the state of Texas. Baylor is private and therefore uses AMCAS.

You will need to submit a general application to each school through these services. You cannot tailor the application for each school. This means that there is one personal statement which goes out to every school. You can adjust the personal statement to each application service, but not to each school. There will be more on this later.

Applications open in May every year and can be submitted either in May or June, depending on the service.

You'll need transcripts for every post-secondary school you attended, demographic information for yourself and your parents, letters of recommendations (LOR) from many different people (look at each school for their LOR requirements), a list of your extracurricular activities with descriptions for each and, of course, your personal statement. The TMDSAS has other essays as part of their primary application as well.

Check the Medical School Application Requirements (MSAR)[3] and College Information Book (CIB)[4] for more information on requirements.

Canada

Most medical schools in Canada have their own application process. Ontario has the Ontario Medical School Application Service (OMSAS), an application service similar to those in the US, which allows you to apply to all of the Ontario medical schools.

---

[3] https://medicalschoolhq.net/msar
[4] https://medicalschoolhq.net/Cib

Most (if not all) Canadian medical schools don't use rolling admissions.

Cost

As of this writing, the primary application costs vary between $150 and $195. TMDSAS is a flat fee of $150 for all schools. AMCAS is $160 and includes one school. Each additional school adds $38 to the total expense. AACOMAS is $195 and also includes one school; each additional school adds another $45.

AACOMAS and AMCAS report the average number of schools being applied to as around 9 and 14, respectively. If students are applying to both MD and DO medical schools, that would mean the average number of schools is 23. That is the high end of the number of schools to which you should plan on applying.

Once you submit your primary application and it is verified, you'll receive secondary applications from most schools. Some schools will be selective about who gets a secondary, but most schools send them to every student, regardless of your ability to get into that school. There is usually a delay before medical schools receive the first batch of applications, so don't expect secondaries immediately if you are applying when the application service first allows you to submit.

Most secondary applications are just extra essays the medical schools want you to include in your application. Most secondary fees are below $100, but I like to tell students to budget $100 per secondary that you need to turn in.

The application process is expensive, which is why you only want to do it once. Be prepared to budget about $5,000 for all of your applications, travel, meals, and wardrobe if you don't already have a suit (for both men and women) in which to interview.

Interviews

The interview season typically opens in August and goes through the beginning of the next year, even as late as April for a few schools. For more information on the medical school interview, check out my other book, *The Premed Playbook: Guide to the Medical School Interview.*[5]

[5] http://www.medschoolinterviewbook.com

When to Start Your Personal Statement

Because writing a great personal statement takes time, I highly recommend starting your first drafts in January of the year you are applying. I don't, however, recommend starting any sooner than that. I've had students reach out to me a couple of years before they were applying, hoping that I could edit their personal statement. You will change a lot as a person and as an applicant as you go through your premed years. Journal your experiences and write your personal statement later. Don't use your personal statement as your journal.

Why should you take so much time to journal your thoughts and then even more time to go through draft after draft of your personal statement? After reading the next chapter, you'll get a much clearer picture as to why the personal statement and good preparation for it are so important.

More Information

Remember, this was just a brief overview of the application process. Be sure to check out each of the individual application service websites for more detailed information about the application process. Check out *The Premed Years*[6] podcast to hear more detailed information about applications.

---

[6] http://www.premedyears.com

CHAPTER 2

WHY YOUR PERSONAL STATEMENT IS IMPORTANT

The application process is a very structured exercise in who can follow directions. You register and open up your primary application. You fill out your demographic information. You fill out information about your family. You enter in all of your grades. You select all the schools that you want to attend and select your letters of recommendations to send to each.

It's not until you get to the extracurricular section that you actually get to start telling your story. The extracurricular section is your first opportunity to show something unique about you—to show what experiences you've had in your life that make you who you are. Even still, with only 700 characters for the AMCAS application, 600 for AACOMAS and 300 for TMDSAS, the extracurricular descriptions don't give you much space to show who you are.

Many students think that the extracurricular descriptions and personal statement have the same function in an application, or even that the extracurriculars could be more important since the total character count is higher if you add them all up. This perception couldn't be further from the truth.

While the extracurriculars are a valuable part of the application, they only tell the reader *what* you have done on your premed journey. The personal statement tells them *why* you are on your journey in the first place.

According to the 2016-2017 AAMC data[1], medical schools reviewed 830,016 applications from 53,042 applicants. Medical schools use your application to figure out if you are a strong enough applicant to be admitted to their school and if you are a unique enough applicant to be part of their class.

Every medical school reviews applications a little bit differently. Some schools will tell you that they read all of their applications. Some schools will filter out applications based on MCAT score or GPA. If your application makes it through the digital shredders, and a member of the Admissions Committee is reading your personal statement, that means your numbers—your GPA and your MCAT score—are probably good enough to be a student at that medical school. Your essay is the next part of the application the reviewer is likely to read.

I think that the personal statement is the most important part of your primary application; it is one of only a few pieces of the application that can help you stand out from the crowd. An Admissions Committee member doesn't form a connection with an MCAT score or a GPA. Those are just numbers on paper. The school may filter out your application based on those two factors, so if the Admissions Committee member is considering your application, they likely won't even care what your scores are at that point. There are even some schools that don't give the reviewer your stats.

If everything else was equal—GPA, MCAT, etc.—your personal statement is likely what will get you an interview over the next student.

I put this quote from Dr. Rivera in the introduction, but thought it would be worth repeating here to highlight to you how crucial the personal statement is:

To be impactful, the personal statement needs to provide Admissions Committees with important insights into why an applicant has chosen to devote his/her life to medicine, and how they hope to improve the

[1] https://www.aamc.org/download/321442/data/factstablea1.pdf

lives of those around them by means of their work as a physician. -
Dean Rivera, Associate Dean of Admission, NYU Medical Center

Dr. Rivera also mentioned that most personal statements seen today don't do this and are not "personal" enough. According to Dean Rivera, with everyone trying to give you input on what should go into a personal statement, usually what you end up with is a "village statement."

In the rest of this book, I'll show you how to brainstorm ideas for your personal statement, how to draft and edit it, and how to finalize the perfect personal statement for **you.** You are the most important piece of the puzzle here. I'm not going to tell you what should go into the personal statement; I'm going to show you how to craft your personal story—the story of why you want to be a doctor and the impact you want to make as one.

Getting to the Interview

The personal statement is the last hurdle between you and your interview. Applications are boring. There are a lot of numbers, transcripts, and information. Your personal statement is the most substantial part in the application in terms of opening up a window to your world so that the reviewer can see who you are and if you are interesting enough to invite for an interview.

Interviews are a very valuable commodity for medical schools. They are time-intensive and cost the school a lot of money to conduct (which is why secondary application fees are so expensive). According to Albert Einstein College of Medicine's 2015-2016 Applicant Guide, they interviewed about 16% of their applicants (1,324 students out of 8,138 applications)[2]. I have found similar numbers on other school's websites.

Your personal statement specifically shows them why you have embarked on this journey and what you hope to accomplish. With that information, schools have a better picture of who you are and if they should invite you for an interview.

[2] https://www.einstein.yu.edu/uploadedFiles/education/md-program/admis/Applicant-Guide-2016.pdf

How Do You Make Yourself Interesting?

The question is: how do you make yourself interesting? I bet if we were talking right now, you'd say, "But, Dr. Gray, I'm not interesting. I haven't done anything 'unique' to stand out." And I would tell you the same thing I tell every student who gives me that same excuse—**you are unique specifically because of who you are!** The life you have led, your parents or guardians, grandparents, aunts, and uncles have all shaped you into who you are. Your friends, your schools, your triumphs, and tragedies all give you a unique lens through which only you look at life. The goal for your applications is to learn how to *show* the reviewer, based on your own personal journey, what you did and how it impacted you to get to this point.

Humans connect with other humans through stories. Readers connect with the stories in your personal statement. It's how we communicate every day. You tell the story of your day to your family when you come home. You connect with the story of the person on the news. You connect with the story of the character in your favorite TV show. Choosing the perfect stories to put in your personal statement can make or break the connection that you can form with an Admissions Committee member.

One of the common ways I describe this journey is with an analogy of a plant. Your journey to medical school began, likely, with the planting of a seed. You were exposed to healthcare through personal illness, family illness, or any of the hundreds of other ways students get their first experience. After that incident, you then watered that seed through volunteering, shadowing, and clinical experiences to prove to yourself that this is what you want to do with your life. This is the journey that you need to tell and the story that must come out.

Look at how this student started her personal statement:

My retinas burned as they filled with flashing red and white lights piercing through the cloud of gravel dust engulfing us. Sitting in my driveway was an ambulance and my mother was inside.

This was her seed. This student then goes on to discuss more of the experience and *why* it played such an important role in her decision to pursue medicine.

If you look at the University of Colorado School of Medicine 2016 data, they received 7,324 applications[3]. They had 7,324 opportunities to read a personal statement, to see if they wanted to have a further discussion with those applicants. If your personal statement isn't interesting enough, memorable enough, or personal enough, then there is a high likelihood that that Admissions Committee is not going to invite you for an interview. In the next chapter, we'll dig into what makes a great personal statement.

You will not be invited for an interview based on your MCAT score and GPA alone. Your MCAT score and GPA may get your application to the top of the list to be reviewed sooner, but a strong personal statement, secondary essays, and the rest of your application are what will get you an interview invite. The Admissions Committee is not going to waste an interview, a limited resource for medical schools, on someone who, judging by their personal statement, isn't interesting enough, or who hasn't shown enough reflection on their journey.

Reflection is going to come up again later, but I want to talk briefly about it here. Too many students just write about the *what* in their personal statement. They highlight a couple of pieces of information from their extracurriculars and flesh them out to fluff up the character count. A great personal statement will tell me the *why* behind their actions and *why* they found them so impactful. Keep an eye out for more discussion about reflection, because it will help you craft a better story.

Is Your Personal Statement Going to Make Up for a Poor GPA or MCAT Score?

Your application is going to be reviewed by each medical school differently. If the medical school you applied to screens applications based on MCAT and GPA, and your scores are lower than their standards, your personal statement is not going to be of any benefit. If your GPA and MCAT score are good enough to get through the first screen, your personal statement can now play a huge role in your ability to be accepted. If you're concerned about writing about your GPA and MCAT score in your personal statement, we'll address that in a later chapter.

---

[3] http://www.ucdenver.edu/academics/colleges/medicalschool/education/community/Matriculation2016/Pages/matricu lation2016.aspx

The Personal Statement vs. Secondary Essays

We'll cover more about secondary essays and how they can help you start thinking about your journey later. For now, it's worth noting that the two types of essays are very different, with different purposes.

The goal of the personal statement, as we have previously discussed, is to show the reader your journey and the experiences that have led you to want to be a physician.

Secondary essays are also very valuable to the Admissions Committee. Some may even say that they are more crucial now that most personal statements aren't accomplishing the goal that they should. Secondary essays are written based on prompts that each school decides they want you to answer. They may ask you to write about diversity, your reasons for applying to their school, obstacles you've overcome, and so much more. Because you are answering a very specific question, usually they are easier to write than just writing about your journey to medicine.

What Now

Now you have a better understanding of why the personal statement is such an essential part of your application. You know that it can make or break your ability to get an interview. With very few interview spots available for so many students, your personal statement is what will help bring your story to life and encourage the Admissions Committee member to want to interview you.

In the next chapter, we're going to dive into what makes a great personal statement.

CHAPTER 3

WHAT MAKES A GREAT PERSONAL STATEMENT

Personal statements are just that. They are *personal*. They are supposed to be about you—about your decision-making journey from the initial inspiration for wanting to be a physician to the experiences that you sought out to confirm that decision.

Admissions Committee members want to know what motivates you to become a physician. They want to make sure you've done your due diligence and that you have reflected on your journey so you know you will like working in the medical field—that you like being around sick people.

Too many students start off down this path because they like watching *Scrubs* or *Grey's Anatomy*. Medicine is not like in TV shows. It's hard. It's draining. It's exhausting. And it's very rewarding. Writing about the experiences that you've had relating to those emotions makes for a great personal statement.

The goal of each and every sentence in your personal statement is to make the reader want to move onto the next sentence. From the first sentence to the last, this is what you want each one to do. Far too often, I start to read a sentence that is trying to do too much, and I want to stop. This is bad.

Here is an example of that from a nontraditional student:

I have been a programmer and computer engineer working in a niche market with great stability. I have built a successful, well-paying career for fifteen years, and I could easily continue on that path until retirement.

That is how the personal statement opened. With that opening, I assumed that this was going to be a résumé-type personal statement and I was immediately turned off. I didn't want to read it anymore. This example was from the student's prior, failed, application. After working on his personal statement together, this is how it opens now:

Watching the smoke rising from the catastrophic explosion at the fertilizer company in Jacksonville, Florida, I felt helpless. I was sitting watching on the news, when what I really wanted to be doing was running toward the scene to help those in need. I knew at this moment that I had made the right decision three years ago to begin on my path to medical school.

Although I currently enjoy a successful, stable career as a programmer and computer engineer, I have chosen to pursue medicine due to a calling to play a more active role in my community.

In this final draft, he leads with a great visual that drew me in and showed me an impactful moment in his life that had solidified in his mind that being a physician was the right path for him. He then went on to mention **briefly** being a programmer and engineer, but quickly brought it back to *why* medicine. In this specific example, he mentioned a more active role in the community. This sort of takeaway isn't always recommended because you can play an active role in your community in any career—but it fits with the rest of his story. Read his final draft, JD Final Draft, in full in Section II of this book.

Here is another example that loses my interest quickly and makes me want to stop reading:

My eight years as an Army officer were the defining experience of my life. I joined ROTC shortly after 9/11, proud to serve the people of the country I loved. The recruiter told me that as an officer I would be in a unique position of influence and responsibility, granted an opportunity to do just what the commercials said: to "be all that you can be."

At the start of a personal statement, I want to feel excited and motivated to read the next line. This example just tells me some basic facts about the student joining ROTC. Why is this important? What am I supposed to take away from this? Those are questions that are floating through my head as I read it. Starting a personal statement in a way that already leaves questions in the reader's head can be detrimental to the experience that you want the reader to have.

I used this example earlier, but I think it's worth including again here. This is a great example of a beginning that draws me to the next line immediately:

My retinas burned as they filled with flashing red and white lights piercing through the cloud of gravel dust engulfing us. Sitting in my driveway was an ambulance and my mother was inside. I could feel the ground that had always felt so steady under my feet begin to tremble.

After reading this, I want to know what happens next, don't you? This is the type of storytelling that draws readers in. This student interviewed with the dean of admissions at a Midwestern allopathic school who told her it was the best personal statement he had ever read. Some may argue that the first sentence crosses over into the creative writing genre. You may be right—but it's only one sentence, so I was okay with it. Her first and final draft can be found in full in Section II—TJ First Draft and TJ Final Draft.

Connection

A good personal statement connects with the reader, elicits emotion from the reader, and makes the reader remember you and your story. You can accomplish this connection by trying to paint a picture for the reader. Help them feel the emotions that you felt. Help them see what you saw. Be careful with this though—many students go a little overboard and turn the personal statement into too much of a creative writing piece. There is a fine balance between too much and just enough.

Look at how this paragraph is written:

One late Saturday evening, an unconscious young woman was being rushed into the emergency department by EMS following a head-on collision on the highway. The nurse was on top of her performing chest compressions on the way to the trauma bay. She appeared to be about my age with dried blood on her bruised face. Shortly after being transferred to the trauma bed, the physician attempted to resuscitate her three times, all of which were unsuccessful. The buzzing of the vitals monitor and the flat rhythm strip was the only sound present. "That's too bad we couldn't bring her back, she was very young."

The student could have easily gone overboard with this paragraph and described the nurse more, given more description of the patient, or even painted a complete picture of the trauma rooms by describing the wall and floor covers, lights, etc. They did a good job of giving enough information to allow the reader to imagine the scenario, without going into unnecessary detail.

The best way to connect with the reader through your personal statement is by *showing* and not *telling*. Don't *tell* the reader you have compassion. *Show* them by telling a story about a situation in which you displayed compassion. Don't *tell* the reader you are passionate about research. *Show* them by painting a picture of you working on your research and the emotions you felt while doing this. We'll talk a lot more throughout the book about *show* vs. *tell*.

Hopefully, you are reading this early on in your journey so I can give you one key piece of advice that will help tremendously with writing your personal statement: **Keep a journal**. We rely too much on our memory to remember experiences from our past—to remember the feelings elicited and the impacts that our actions had on other people. Keeping a journal and journaling after each of your extracurricular activities will give you a huge advantage when preparing your applications.

The Impact

A great personal statement doesn't just list your experiences. If you write that you volunteered at a free clinic, this doesn't set you apart because thousands of other applicants have likely also volunteered at a free clinic. You need to write about the impact of that experience on you as a person and on you as a future physician. This is where keeping a journal is very important. Don't rely on your memory to remember experiences from several years ago. After each experience that you have, keep track of what was impactful for you. When you are ready to start drafting your personal statement, you can look back at these notes for inspiration.

Part of writing about that impact is your ability to *reflect* on what you've done instead of just writing *about* what you've done. You need to start with your *why* in mind. There is a great TED Talk by author Simon Sinek titled, *How Great Leaders Inspire Action*[1]. It is based on his book *Start with Why*. If you can reflect back on your experiences and show the reader *why* each of those experiences has influenced your journey, you will rise above the superficial aspects of just writing about your experiences. This is memorable. This makes for a great personal statement.

When you are done with your personal statement, you should have shown the reader examples of experiences that you've had that have made an impact on you. Tell me the story of a patient you interacted with that left you saying, "YES! This is why I want to be a doctor." There is a big difference between *showing* the reader those emotions and just *telling* them that you went through the motions of getting the experience.

[1] https://www.ted.com/talks/simon_sinek_how_great_leaders_inspire_action

Good Takeaways

Just because you have told me a story of shadowing or interacting with a patient doesn't mean you're done. You also have to tell me *why* that experience was worth writing about. What is your takeaway? Put another way, how did the experience impact your decision to continue down the path to becoming a physician?

Look at this example from a draft:

In another of my shadowing experiences, the surgeon allowed me to scrub in to assist in minor roles during a cesarean section. Moments before making the first incision, he leaned over to me and asked if I am okay around blood. I assured him I am, and he began. He asked me to hold the retractor during the procedure. I will always remember the surprising wave of amniotic fluid that covered my hand and wrist when the amniotic sac was broken. This exciting event was quickly outdone by the emergence of new life that was rushed to the mother's arms.

What's the takeaway here? Did the student feel amazed at being able to care for someone? Was he in awe of bringing life into this world? Did he want to continue this feeling in his career? Without proper reflection, this statement doesn't tell me anything.

Here is another example of a student trying to give me a takeaway but failing to give me enough information:

Watching the dynamic that develops between the patient with his or her family members, and seeing the sacrifices they are willing to make drive me to continue to push myself and provide me a constant reminder of why I must do so.

Must do what? The "dynamic" between patients and physicians is unique, but you can have dynamics with people in other career fields. There needed to be more than just "dynamics."

Here is a strong takeaway from a student who was volunteering in the emergency department:

Volunteering in the emergency department, there was one night a person came to the front desk saying her husband was having chest pains in the car. I grabbed a wheelchair and quickly went to the car. I helped him get in the car and brought him straight to a room for diagnosis and care by the trained staff members. While being proud to provide a part of the service to this patient, I wanted to be able to help in a more important role.

"I wanted to be able to help in a more important role." You may think that this sentence is too simple to be impactful, but it is. Simple is good. It's easy to read. It tells me what the student is thinking, and it definitely points the student in the direction of becoming a physician.

Here's another example of a great takeaway from a student after telling a story about needing healthcare in a foreign country as a traveler.

I had experienced the powerful impact an empathetic caregiver can have on a patient. I wanted to provide that comfort and care for others; to pass on the compassion that was shown to me in a time of need.

This is a very straightforward takeaway. It doesn't need to be fancy. It just needs to show me that you have thought about your experience and you know how it affected you and why you are using that as motivation to move forward.

Reflection is one of the most important parts of the personal statement. It shows the Admissions Committee that you're not just going through the motions of checking off boxes, but instead, you are gaining experiences that are showing you that this is the right path for you. You need to reflect so that you can create the best takeaways. And you need great takeaways to explain your journey to the Admissions Committee.

Before we dive into what to write about, and more on reflection, I want to give you an idea of how the Admissions Committee may review your personal statement. That's what we'll explore next.

CHAPTER 4

HOW YOUR PERSONAL STATEMENT IS REVIEWED

Before I show you what to write about and how to start writing your personal statement, I want to explain what Admissions Committees may be looking at in your personal statement. This is one of the most common questions students ask: What does the Admissions Committee want to read about? There has to be some secret checklist or algorithm they are using, right?

Unfortunately, the answer is yes and no. There is no perfect personal statement template. We've already talked about how every student is unique and that you need to tell **your** story. But, that doesn't mean that Admissions Committee members aren't looking into what you are writing about or that they aren't trying to read into you or your personality from the stories you tell.

The AAMC has a list of 15 core competencies[1] for entering medical students that medical schools use to help them determine which students to invite for

[1] https://medicalschoolhq.net/aamccompetencies

an interview and who to accept. Admissions Committees are looking at your personal statement to determine if you demonstrate some of these competencies and, therefore, if they want to invite you for an interview.

The core competencies are broken down into four categories: interpersonal, intrapersonal, thinking and reasoning, and science. While these core competencies have been developed to help guide admissions to medical school, you should not use this as an exhaustive list of what you need to discuss in your personal statement.

Rather, here are the competencies which I think are the most relevant to the personal statement. Note that these are not all of the competencies listed by the AAMC. These are not provided so you have a template for your personal statement, but so you can understand how medical schools may be evaluating you while they are reading your applications and, later, during your interview day.

Interpersonal Competencies

Service Orientation: Service Orientation should be very easy to show in your personal statement and your application as a whole. The stories that you tell will show that you can put others' needs before yourself—that you can respond to other people's needs, feelings, and emotions. Your extracurricular activity list and your personal statement will demonstrate this competency. You can write about whom you positively affected with your volunteering. You should show the impact that you made on the people you were serving.

Cultural Competence: Cultural Competence can be shown through stories of your experiences that involve interacting with or working with a diverse set of patients. With the U.S. becoming more and more diverse, you will be treating people from all walks of life and you will need to demonstrate an understanding of socio-cultural factors that affect you and your patients.

Teamwork: You can discuss teamwork with stories of working in a group to help a patient. If you have a story about teamwork that is significant enough to make the cut for your personal statement, you need to show how you played a part in that team. Demonstrating the ability to work in a team is paramount to healthcare in the future. Each healthcare team involves many different people, all working together to provide each patient with the best care possible; these include physicians from multiple specialties, nurses, social workers, and physical therapists, just to name a few.

Interpersonal Competencies

Resilience and Adaptability: Most personal statements seem to revolve around this competency. Writing about a time you were sick or injured and coming back from that determined to become a physician is a classic example of resilience and adaptability. Overcoming a parent's illness and supporting a family is also a common example. Writing about an abnormally poor semester and what you learned can also be used to show this competency. We all adapt and have to bounce back in our day-to-day lives. Select a story if it's impactful enough to bring your resilience to the fore.

Capacity for Improvement: Capacity for Improvement could be shown in a story about your journey to becoming a physician. From the moment you learned about medicine and becoming a physician, to the day that you are writing your personal statement, you have hopefully surrounded yourself with experiences of improvement. Writing about the key experiences that you have encountered and how you improved as a premed is a great discussion topic for a personal statement.

Thinking and Reasoning Competencies

Written Communication: Written Communication is pretty straightforward. How well you communicate in your personal statement will give the Admissions Committee an idea of your competency in this area.

Summary

Knowing what the Admissions Committee is looking for in a student is important and trying to highlight your experiences to show your competencies in these areas is also important, but you don't want to cross the line and write a personal statement just for the Admissions Committee. As soon as you start writing a personal statement for the Admissions Committee, that's when it is no longer a *personal* statement. You need to tell your story. You need to tell the Admissions Committee member–that person reading your personal statement–why you want to be a physician and what experiences you have had along the way that have guided you down that path. We're going to delve into what to write about in the next chapter.

CHAPTER 5

WHAT TO WRITE ABOUT

Whether you are a 21-year-old traditional premed applying to medical school, or you're a 45-year-old nontraditional premed looking to change careers, you've likely had a lot of experiences in your life that have made an impact on you.

There are two questions you need to ask yourself. First, "What was the first time in my life that I questioned if being a physician was right for me?" Second, "What are the most impactful experiences that have continued to strengthen my desire to become a physician?" Impactful can mean different things to different students, so you just need to look back on your experiences and try to remember which ones mean the most to you.

Your personal statement is meant to provide the Admissions Committee with the reasons behind your journey to medical school while also showing who you are. You're embarking on a career in the medical field, in which about half of physicians are burnt out[1]. Many physicians are unhappy with the pay they

[1] https://www.medscape.com/sites/public/lifestyle/2017

receive, with the hours they work, and the many different aspects and struggles of medicine. Knowing this, why are you deciding to enter this field? I'm not telling you this to scare you away. I'm sharing this information because it's true. (For a little more info on physicians and their careers, check out my podcast, Specialty Stories at specialtystories.com.)

At the end of the personal statement, the reader should have a clear picture of who you are and your reasons for wanting to be a physician. It should be clear why you want to be a physician and not necessarily something else like a nurse, physician assistant (PA), or social worker.

Look at these bullet points from a personal statement:

- *It became clear to me that I yearned to serve others beyond the classroom, in a more vital role.*
- *A lack of access to care has always existed in our neighborhood, the chaos simply amplified the dilemma of living in a medically underserved community.*
- *I saw firsthand how formidable the barriers to treatment were in St. Louis*

These takeaways don't tell me the student wants to be a physician; just that he wants to make a difference. Read his full personal statement, SR Early Draft, by downloading free, extra essays at personalstatementbook.com/bonusessays.

Look at this example from a student:

Due to my experiences being hospitalized and overcoming English language barriers, I am passionate about being a "cheerleader" for others.

What does being a "cheerleader" for others mean? It doesn't say she wants to be a physician. In my mind, it's **not** saying that she *needs* to be a physician. I think it's telling the reader that she wants to support people. It doesn't specifically say patients, just "others." Don't muddy the waters of your personal statement with obscure statements like these. It will have the reader second-guessing *why* you are doing this.

Being clear about why you want to be a physician includes being clear about starting to explore the career as well. Many students just jump straight into shadowing a physician or volunteering at the hospital and don't write about much else before that. In these cases, I'm always left wondering why they started to explore that interest in the first place.

Here is an example of one student just jumping right in without giving the reader much insight into her backstory:

> *But as I got older, I realized I didn't want to center my life around politics and that I had no desire to overcome stage fright. However, my interest in the well-being of others and love for scientific knowledge only increased. So I set my eyes on the goal – study Biology, get that degree and jump right into medical school.*

This brief statement about jumping right into medical school doesn't give me enough understanding of the student's reasons for wanting to be a physician. This gives the reader pause, causing them to question if the student really knows about that with which she is getting involved.

You have to give a little bit more of the backstory into *why* you first started shadowing, or *why* your passion is medicine and being a physician.

Reflection

I talked briefly about reflection in the What Makes a Great Personal Statement chapter when I was explaining how strong takeaways are essential for a great personal statement. We're going to look at that idea a little deeper here.

Look up the definition for reflection, and you'll see that it means: "serious thought or consideration." For every action that you've taken, every experience that you've had, you should give some serious thought *and* consideration into how it has either made you want to be a physician or not want to do something else.

The only way to find the answer to *why medicine* is through reflection. You have to understand what your goals are, and you have to reflect upon how your journey is leading you there. When you are looking through the experiences you have had along the way, and you reflect upon why you're thinking about putting one specific experience in your personal statement, you have to ask yourself:

"What is it about this experience that has further strengthened my desire and drive to be a physician?"

Reflecting upon your journey should lead you to ask some tough questions. It will help you avoid writing about trivial experiences from your past that *you* think are important but that might not be so interesting to the reader. Playing doctor as a child, and knowing that that is what you wanted to do with your life is **not** your reason for becoming a physician. Having a parent who is a physician is **not** your reason for becoming a physician. Your experiences *after* those moments in your life give you the memories that you can then reflect on to build your story.

A lot of students write about how they have shadowed and witnessed physicians doing amazing things for patients. They explain how they want to do that for patients too. This is very superficial. It's obvious. It doesn't offer the **why** behind it. This is where reflection comes into play.

This is why it's very tricky to write about experiences that you've witnessed instead of personal interactions. The emotions behind personal experiences are so much more powerful, which means that reflecting upon them gives you the answers right away.

Look at this example from a student writing about his experience shadowing:

The most impactful moment I had shadowing was with a palliative care physician. The patient was nearing the end of a battle with cancer but had not yet come to terms with her reality. I watched the physician artfully balance the severity of the patient's condition with compassion and empathy. I was struck by the physician's rapport; how honest, yet gentle, he remained. It really demonstrated how physicians can dignify their patients in the most difficult situations.

All that this tells the reader is that the student enjoyed witnessing the doctor-patient relationship. The takeaway is that the doctor demonstrated dignifying patients. This was probably a great moment for the student, but the story could be much more powerful if he wrote about *his* interaction with the patient.

Now, let's look at an example of a student writing about a personal experience with a patient and how that interaction drives her to pursue becoming a physician:

The first day I came into Jane's room, she motioned for me to sit down on a hard plastic chair. We began chatting, and within an hour, she told me about how her husband had died, followed by her son, then followed the murder of her daughter. I was astounded. After she told me, she looked out the window and said, "You don't think about it too much. Only when the weather is cloudy." That day, Jane exemplified what I have seen in many hospice patients. They are vulnerable, candid, and often resilient. They leave me wanting to do everything I can to ease their burdens.

Because the student is interacting directly with the patient, her reflection on this experience is much more compelling. Notice that this student didn't say, "They leave me wanting to do everything to spend more time with them." Or, "They leave me wanting to continue building a relationship with them." She said, "ease their burdens." Building relationships and spending time can be something a nurse, social worker, or other healthcare team member can do. While "easing burdens" isn't specifically the job of a physician, it's not a giant leap to assume that the student is writing about being a physician.

If you truly believe a time when you observed something was your most powerful moment, and you think you simply have to write about it, go ahead. Just know that it probably isn't as powerful of a story as a direct interaction with a patient. As an aside, it definitely is okay to write about the impact of observing in your extracurricular descriptions.

The rest of this chapter will give you some ideas of topics on which you can reflect.

Helping People and Loving Science

Too many students write about wanting to help people. I took an Uber once and asked the driver how his day was going. "I'm having a great day; I'm helping people!" I laughed to myself because his response is why I always make this argument. **You can help people in any career.**

Students will then try to mix in helping people and the love of science, but again, you can use science and helping people in many different careers in healthcare. You could be a physical therapist or a psychologist. You could be a nurse or a PA. Stay far away from these statements as reasons for why you want to be a doctor. They are part of it, but not the reasons for your adventure.

Bad Experience with Physicians

Believe it or not, I see this a lot. A physician treated a student, or their family, poorly and that motivated the student to be a physician. Don't write about this. I talk more about why in the *What to Avoid* chapter.

Did You Ever Take a Break?

Did you ever take a hiatus from the premed path? It's okay to include this in a personal statement. It shows you've done some reflection. It shows that you've been challenged once (or more) before and that when the toughness of medical school, or residency, hits you, you aren't going to run away. This part of the personal statement shouldn't be long, but if you can work it into your story, it will show who you are much better than just ignoring it.

Nontraditional Students

Refection is where nontraditional students can knock it out of the park. If you are coming from another career field or if you had to take some time off due to poor grades or other reasons, you likely have very strong reasons for changing course and coming "back" to medicine as a goal.

See how this student wrote about coming back to being a premed after another career in a different field:

> *Thus, life events and fear of the academic rigor in medical school forged a path away from healthcare; yet, I never forgot the experiences from my formative years. They are what fuel my renewed passion to be a physician today. It's why I have gotten involved in research related to obesity and diabetes, seeking out potential therapeutic targets to manage the downstream effects of obesity.*

Earlier in the personal statement, he discussed his other career briefly before going into the initial reasons for his interest in medicine. You can see his full personal statement, NL Final Draft, by downloading free, extra essays at personalstatementbook.com/bonusessays.

Because this student describes walking away from his earlier dreams, working in corporate America, and then having an experience that brought him back, he is able to show the Admissions Committee that he has reflected on his journey.

You don't have to be a nontraditional student to reflect on your journey, though. Don't think that you should purposefully not apply to medical school, go out into the working world, and then come back to medicine to show you have reflected as well. (Yes, I have been asked this, so I need to put it in here.)

Drawing Upon Your Extracurricular Experiences

Looking back at the chapter on why your personal statement is important, you'll remember what I told you about extracurriculars. Looking ahead, I must reassert that your personal statement shouldn't just be a list of your extracurriculars.

I'll assume here that you didn't just "check off" some boxes and participate in extracurriculars "just because." Hopefully, you have strengthened your resolve to become a physician through some of your extracurriculars.

One of your experiences could be the key to why you want to be a doctor. Just because it's an extracurricular activity, you don't *need* to leave it out of your personal statement. It's *how* you put it in that makes all the difference in the world.

Here is an example of an extracurricular experience that belongs in the personal statement:

In my journey to discover if medicine is truly my calling, I volunteered as a friendly visitor for the Mental Health Association of State County. Through the program, I befriended a blind senior citizen who struggles with various health issues, among which is depression. Often, my presence and help alleviated some of the pain and loneliness he suffered, according to him, but there was limited help I could provide for him as a friend visiting him once or twice a week. Although I was armed with a friendly and empathetic demeanor, it was never going to equal the treatment that a physician could offer him. Therefore, working with him in depth helped me to appreciate the value and the necessity of psychiatric help. In addition, witnessing his struggles and triumphs while battling with depression intensified my desire to become a doctor to better understand mental disorders and to help patients suffering like my friend.

This is a great example because the overall message was clear. She had a strong takeaway that the experience strengthened her desire to be a physician. She also had some statements that she didn't need. Telling the reader that you have a "friendly and empathetic demeanor" is the student trying to sell the reader skills. Another tip is that if you are struggling to find some extra characters in your personal statement; you can remove the names of the places you are volunteering.

Talking About Specialties

A very common question is whether or not students should write about the specific career in which they are interested. Some advisors will tell you to avoid it. Some, like myself, will tell you that as long as you tell your story well enough, and it revolves around a specific specialty, it can be okay.

Out of the hundreds of personal statements I have read, I can only think of two or three in which the student specifically wrote about a specialty effectively.

At this point in the process, your goal is to get into medical school. At this point, trying to work in your specialty preference is taking up extra space that could be better utilized on another point.

The other very simple reason not to do this is that, once in medical school, most students usually decide to pursue a different career than what they arrived hoping to practice.

Brainstorming Ideas

The following is a list (in no way complete) of what your initial exposure (the planting of the seed) to medicine may have been, including some common experiences that lead students down the premed path:

- personal healthcare journey (cancer survivor, autoimmune disease, hospital stay, sports injury) (Read more about this in the *Red Flags, Disabilities, and Other Events* chapter.)
- family healthcare journey (parent's cancer battle, sibling's mental health battle, healthcare access struggles, family member's battle with addiction)
- birth of a child
- relationship with a mentor
- family member in healthcare
- being a helpless bystander during a medical emergency

Using Secondary Essay Prompts

Looking at secondary essay prompts is another way to start understanding yourself better to determine what you want to write about. The secondary applications come after medical schools receive your primary application. These applications usually have essay prompts asking you to write on topics such as obstacles that you've overcome, your motivations for becoming a physician, or your most memorable clinical experience. Thinking about these essay prompts, reflecting on your journey, and starting to write responses to these prompts may help you get an idea of your motivations and help you formulate what you want to write about in your personal statement.

Here are some essay prompts to help you think about your journey and what you may want to write about:

Nontraditional Student or Student with Possible Academic Difficulties

- Have you had any lapse of two years or greater in taking full-time college-level coursework?
- Please provide below any additional information you believe is important in evaluating your application (e.g., additional coursework, problems with academic record; disadvantaged, etc.).

Red Flags (we'll dive more into red flags in another chapter)
- Describe any academic performance issues you have experienced and how you got back on course. (This prompt can help you address any red flags that you may have in your application.)
- If you've received a grade of C or less in a class, please explain.

Initial Motivations for Being a Physician or Experiences that have Strengthened Your Desire to be One (Planting of the Seed)
- Please describe a volunteer or service activity that played a large part in your decision to become a physician.
- Describe in detail the three extracurricular activities or experiences that have been most influential in leading you to a career in medicine.
- Please write about things in your background that have been important to your development or that have been challenging to you on your path to a career in medicine. These could include your socioeconomic status, culture, race, ethnicity, sexual orientation, sexual identity, and work or life experiences. **Explain how these have influenced your goals and preparation for a career in medicine.**
- Have you lived in communities which are medically underserved, or where the majority of the population is economically and/or educationally disadvantaged? (And, to provide the info you need for a good personal statement, how did this add to your desire to be a physician?)
- Have you worked with medically underserved, economically disadvantaged and/or educationally disadvantaged populations? (And, to provide the info you need for a good personal statement, how did this add to your desire to be a physician?)
- What has been your most significant patient encounter?

The Future

- What do you see as the most likely practice scenario for your future medical career?
- Briefly, describe the community you anticipate practicing medicine in post-residency.
- What are your future professional aspirations?

Summary

You may read this and be disappointed to learn that many students have the same story as you. During a Premed Years podcast interview with Michigan State University College of Osteopathic Medicine's Dean, Dr. Strampel, he stated that about 80% of the personal statements they receive follow the same storyline.

In the chapter about how to be unique, I discussed why this isn't something that you should worry about. There are dozens, if not hundreds, of popular books and movies that follow the same storyline, yet they are all different.

As long as you stick to the goal of the *personal* statement—telling your *personal* journey—your essay will be good. Then you just need to follow along with the rest of the advice in this book to make it great.

CHAPTER SIX

HOW TO START WRITING YOUR PERSONAL STATEMENT

I f you're like most people, the sheer effort involved in learning about what to write about, drafts, editing, and everything else that goes into the personal statement is likely preventing you from starting.

After reading through some of the basics on how to get started with your personal statement, you will have the knowledge to dive in either right now, or as soon as it's time, based on when you are applying.

How Others Started Their Personal Statement

I reached out to several students and asked for their comments on how they went about starting to put their personal statements together. The following are their comments:

I started by reading 10-20 personal statement examples to get a sense of how other students approached the personal statement. I also talked with Dr. Gray and brainstormed the main details of my personal story. After I wrote an initial draft, I set aside time each week to revise. I wrote 1-2 drafts per week and had Dr. Gray read and revise my drafts. The entire process lasted about 3 months. – SH

The hardest part was just getting it started. I wrote a draft. Then I waited a few days, came back to it, made a bunch of edits, and then saved it again. I saved every draft, this way if I deleted a story, I could always add it back in again (copy and paste from a prior draft). Knowing that any edit I made was never permanent allowed me to make drastic changes. This prevented me from getting too attached to any aspect of my statement and really helped me tease out the best aspects of my drafts. After several drafts, I started asking people for feedback (both proofreading for grammatical errors and suggestions on content). This step is so important! Sometimes you need a new set of eyes to look at your essay to make sure that your thoughts are clear and your grammar is correct. – JW

Like many nontraditional students, I was really struggling with how I was going to fit my long, winding journey and experiences into such a small essay. I had so many experiences I wanted to convey, and I would literally lay awake at night trying to decide which ones I wanted to tell, and how I wanted to tie them together. Every time I sat down and tried to write however, I would start to second guess myself. I wrote about what I thought an Admissions Committee would want to hear, rather than the story I wanted to tell. I was never happy with what came out, so I would throw it all out.

My wife actually suggested I take the "write drunk, edit sober" advice literally, so I had a few drinks and sat down at the keyboard. With my inhibitions gone, I poured my unfiltered heart and thoughts onto the screen. It was long, and very rough around the edges, but it was an honest representation of my journey and my desire to practice medicine. The next day I sat down to edit, and with the drunken foundation I had laid, I was finally able to get my first draft completed. – DM

Before I wrote my first draft, I reflected on my entire life and the things that were important to me. From there, I thought about which of those had to do with medicine and then determined what the linkages between those things were. I then thought about examples that illustrated that linkage and wrote about some highlight experiences to support my final decision to pursue medicine. – AS

When to Start Writing Your Personal Statement

Applications open in May and June each year for those planning to start medical school the following year. Knowing that you need to apply early, your personal statement should be done by this time.

Start working on an outline of your personal statement and thinking about the stories you want to tell around January, and you'll probably have plenty of time to go through several drafts of your essay, as well as get feedback and take the necessary breaks to return to your work with fresh eyes.

How Many Drafts Should I Write?

This one is very specific to each student. It depends on how good your first draft is at telling the story of why you want to be a doctor. I've seen students do it in as little as three or four drafts. Some students kept polishing even after 12 drafts.

The key takeaway from this should be that it takes more than just one draft. Be prepared to write around six. If you can do it with fewer drafts, great. If it takes you more, that's okay too.

What I don't want you to do is start your personal statement late and either have it delay your application or for you to hurry through it to get your application submitted as soon as you can. The personal statement is too important to rush. Choose a date in January of the year you are planning to apply. This is when you will start to outline your personal statement. Mark this date on your calendar now.

The Essay Prompts

If you read the *AMCAS Instruction Manual*[1], and I suggest you do, you'll read this about the personal statement:

Use the Personal Comments Essay as an opportunity to distinguish yourself from other applicants. Consider and write your Personal Comments Essay carefully; many admission committees place significant weight on the essay.

Here are some questions that you may want to consider while writing the essay:
- *Why have you selected the field of medicine?*
- *What motivates you to learn more about medicine?*
- *What do you want medical schools to know about you that hasn't been disclosed in other sections of the application?*

In addition, you may wish to include information such as:
- *Unique hardships, challenges, or obstacles that may have influenced your educational pursuits*
- *Comments on significant fluctuations in your academic record that are not explained elsewhere in your application*

The AACOMAS Instruction Manual[2] asks you to:

Write a brief statement expressing your motivation or desire to become a DO.

The TMDSAS[3] prompt for the personal statement is very straightforward:

Explain your motivation to seek a career in medicine. Be sure to include the value of your experiences that prepare you to be a physician.

You'll notice that none of these prompts ask you to write about why you will be a good doctor. All of them want you to comment on **why you want to be a doctor.**

[1] https://medicalschoolhq.net/amcasguide
[2] https://medicalschoolhq.net/aacomasinstructions
[3] https://www.tmdas.com/medical/section_Overview.html

I really like how the TMDSAS prompt asks you for the *value* of your experiences; they want you to reflect on the experience, not just tell the reader about it. For more on this, refer back to the chapter about what makes a personal statement great.

Apps to Outline

There are many ways to start outlining a personal statement, or any other essay, for that matter. Some students like good old pen and paper. Some prefer more high-tech options.

I'm a fan of mind mapping. If you're not familiar with this tool, it's a way to organize information visually. It's kind of like a bulleted outline, but much more usable for the way my mind works. I can move bubbles around and draw connections between different thoughts. There are free and paid mind mapping apps out there. I like MindNode, but it's macOS/iOS only. A simple Google search will help you find something compatible with your device.

If you're more of a list person, a normal outlining tool or any word processor can get the job done. There is a free online app called Workflowy that works well for organizing thoughts in a list.

How to Prepare for Your First Draft

Unfortunately, most students open up their software or notebook and just stare at a blank screen/paper. They think about everything they need to go through and get overwhelmed by trying to figure out what to write about. Then they just open up Facebook or Netflix instead.

Download our free checklist to help you start gathering ideas for your first draft by going to personalstatementbook.com/checklist.

Here is what one student came up with when he was brainstorming:

- *addressing college failures, responsibility, maturity, focus,*
- *working as a scribe*
- *mentorship by physicians*
- *path to want to be a physician, came together gradually, intersection of interest in nutrition/wellness, biochemistry and prevention*
- *role as personal trainer, found great satisfaction in using my knowledge in an applied fashion to help people on a personal level*

- *mention osteopathic medicine???*
- *my path to applying, postbac, struggles, what I learned about myself.*

The goal of outlining your personal statement is to give yourself a direction for when you start putting words to paper. If you go in with a plan, you are less likely to ramble on through the essay and end up somewhere totally different from where you wanted to be. Remember that the goal of the essay is to write about why you want to be a physician. Try thinking about some of the most powerful moments in your journey (usually two or three) that left you wanting to do this more than anything else.

Remember that the goal of the personal statement is to tell the Admissions Committee about your journey to becoming a physician. How did you first get interested in medicine? What have you been doing to explore that interest? What are you hoping to do with your career? Those should be the main points to outline. If you've had some major red flags, then those should be included as well. I'll explain more about red flags later.

Leave This Out of Your Brainstorming

There will be a full "what to avoid in your personal statement" chapter later, but I want to address one common, huge mistake that students make when brainstorming ideas. I've mentioned it once already, but I need to do it again.

Do not, for a second, think that you have to tell the reader that you like science and are dedicated to helping people. These ideas do not belong in your personal statement. I'm not just saying that you should avoid specifically saying, "I like science and want to help people." You should definitely avoid that. What I'm saying is that you should also avoid trying to incorporate those specific themes into your personal statement.

This student jumped right in with one of the most clichéd statements he could make:

The first time I said I wanted to be a physician, I was 14 years old. My geometry teacher had asked me what my goals were after high school. I told him I wanted to be a doctor, and he asked me what my motivation was. My response, reflective of my age, maturity, and lack of understanding of what being a physician constituted: I merely "liked science."

Obviously, the student knew this was cliché, which is why he prefaced it the way he did, but it still doesn't belong in the personal statement.

Here's another one from a student who forced in the science statement in a draft:

My interest in science began in elementary school, but that interest shifted to medicine in junior high when my grandfather started to face some serious health issues.

The feedback I gave him was to delete the science comment and start with medicine.

One student tried to sneak in helping people with this comment:

People are another passion of mine.

I think you can guess that I suggested she remove that statement.

Your First Draft

Earnest Hemingway once famously said, "write drunk, edit sober." I love these words for helping students start their personal statement. Being a premed, you are likely a highly analytical type-A student, and you want to make sure everything is perfect when you're putting pen to paper; or fingers to keyboard, as it is nowadays.

Unfortunately, that's not how good first drafts come about. A good first draft needs to be uninhibited, which is where the *write drunk* part comes in. You need to just spill your thoughts and get your fingers moving as fast as you can, without hesitation. You need to get all of your ideas out of your head without editing them inside your head beforehand. This is the number one killer of great ideas when it comes to writing. Don't let your self-doubt or self-editing cause you to miss out on something great.

Ernest Hemingway also famously said, "The first draft of anything is sh*t." That is where most premed students get scared. Perfection is what you shoot for every time, from tests to essays. Everything that you have done to this point is probably a great work of art, and you are scared to create something that is less than that, but that is what your first draft needs to be. It needs to be sh*t.

Your first draft is **not** the final product. It is actually far from it. It takes a good two months—three months even—plus a half-dozen or more drafts to make a polished personal statement. Too many students cut corners and try to go from the first draft to the final draft in one step. That's just not how it works. One of the students I worked with recently submitted her first draft to me on January 24th. Her final draft, number 13, was done on April 2nd.

Your first draft doesn't have to be cohesive. It doesn't have to be one idea. Your first draft can be 10,000 characters of rambling mess. It's just your first draft. Don't worry if it's over the word count. Don't worry if it doesn't make sense to anyone else. Don't look at grammar, spelling, or punctuation. Just get the thoughts and ideas out of your head.

When I'm teaching at the medical school, I tell the students every time: "this is a safe place. Practice what you want to try in here, so I can give you feedback before you try it with a real patient." Your first draft is the same. You don't have to show it to anyone. You have my permission to make it as terrible as possible. I won't judge you. No one will. The goal is to get it done.

Some students that I've talked to have taken this idea to *write drunk* quite literally and have had a few drinks before they write their first draft of their personal statement. They say it helps. I'm not advocating drinking, and if you are underage, then definitely stay away. Luckily we live in a technological era, and there are apps to assist you achieve the same results sober. These apps prevent you from deleting or editing anything, which is great.

Apps

One of these apps is called Ernest, which, obviously, is named after Ernest Hemingway. There is also an app called Flowstate, which will delete everything you have done if you stop typing before the time you designate. Now, I think that's a little bit crazy, but it is one way of hacking your way to a first draft. It prevents you from stopping and thinking. You just need to type and get it out of your head. There are several apps like this, but ultimately, what it comes down to, is getting the information out of your head. *I Love Your Story* at ilys.com is also a useful app. You tell it how many words you want to write, and it won't let you edit until you get to that number. You can't even see what you wrote until you get there. It really gets your mind moving.

Dictate

One of the strategies that I recommend for students, especially for those who have a long commute, is to use an app called Rev[1]. Rev allows you to dictate your thoughts into your phone or computer. The app then uploads that dictation to a transcriptionist who will provide you with a transcribed document in a day. This is a perfect way to create your first draft because, when you're speaking, it is hard to edit your thoughts as they come out. You just start talking and don't stop. You then take that transcript and start moving and editing and massaging your message from there. It's a great way to write a first draft. It's actually how I did the first draft of this book.

The main takeaway here is that you just need to start. Stop thinking about it and just start writing (or dictating). You don't have to submit everything that you've written in your application; you just need to submit that final, polished draft. Don't be scared to create those initial sh*t drafts so that you can get to the good stuff that is in your head.

Editing and Iterating

I think the editing and iterating process is too robust to include in this chapter, so I'll have a whole chapter dedicated to that. In that chapter, I'll cover who should be giving you feedback, what questions you should be asking, and how you should be improving your personal statement each step of the way.

What's next?

Now that you understand what to write about and how to start writing your personal statement, it's time to go further into other aspects of the personal

[1] https://www.rev.com

statement, including writing about red flags, how your personal statement will be reviewed, and so much more.

CHAPTER SEVEN

WRITING ABOUT RED FLAGS, DISABILITIES, AND OTHER EVENTS

In the last chapter, I gave you a lot of information about how to craft a story around your journey to medicine. Part of that journey may include other aspects of your life that you think you want to include. Some of those will be important to write about, and others I would recommend leaving out. That's what I'll cover here.

Red Flags

Some advisors will advise you to write about your red flags, and some will tell you to avoid them. Let's start by defining what a red flag is. If you've been arrested, for anything, at any time, that will likely be a red flag. If you've been dismissed from an academic institution, that is probably a red flag. If you have a terrible semester sandwiched inbetween great semesters, that could also be a red flag. If you have negative trends in your grades, meaning you started poorly your first two years but did well at the end, or you did well at the beginning and dropped off towards graduation, that could be a red flag.

A lower than average MCAT score is not a red flag. A lower than average GPA is not a red flag. Students often like to discuss those stats, but the Admissions Committee is not so concerned with these numbers. If your stats are bad enough that you're doing a postbac, then you may want to consider that, but just briefly.

A lack of certain extracurriculars, like shadowing, clinical experience, or research could be a red flag, but it will be hard to explain in your personal essay why you didn't do these obvious prerequisites.

If you are an introvert, have a fear of talking to people, or a fear of confrontation, these are personality traits and not red flags. I wouldn't bring any of these up. I wouldn't write about being scared of blood. You'd be surprised how fast you grow past that during medical school.

Ultimately, it's up to you to decide what could be a red flag in your application.

Here is My Take on Including Red Flags in Your Personal Statement

If you've had significant red flags on your journey, they need to be in your personal statement, but *they should not* ***be*** *your personal statement*. Your personal statement still needs to show the Admissions Committee why you want to be a doctor. It still needs to show that you've reflected on your journey. Going on and on about some of your struggles will cause you to lose the ability to convey the proper message. The reader will not find those aspects intriguing enough to invite you for an interview.

This is one of the largest mistakes that students make when discussing a red flag—they go too in depth about their red flags and don't tell their main story well enough. That is: their story about why they want to be a physician. This turns the personal statement into one long laundry list of problems and doesn't tell enough stories about your journey, your motivations, or your passions.

Why would an Admissions Committee want to invite you for an interview if all that they see in your personal statement is a list of reasons why you were rejected from school, kicked out of school, struggled in school, struggled on the MCAT, or reasons why you were arrested? There is too much risk and not enough upside when a personal statement airs your dirty laundry like that.

The goal is to offer just enough information to satisfy them that you are aware of a possible concern in your application, and to provide just enough of a story for them to want to ask you more about it when you come for an interview.

One student I worked with had a gap in her education in high school after delaying graduation and starting college because of the health of her father.

Here is the story she first drafted:

During my senior year, when my mother's health significantly worsened, I made the decision to postpone my high school graduation and college matriculation. Though I regret the hasty way in which I went about this decision, I am grateful for the path it took me down. Unfortunately, my undergraduate GPA is negatively affected by dual-enrollment classes I took during that time, lowering it to a 3.69 as calculated by AMCAS from a 3.93 (my cumulative GPA at State University, which allows for repeated courses to be excluded from GPA calculations). With that said, I am absolutely grateful for the decision I made to postpone my college education, as I returned to school with a vigor and motivation that can only be found intrinsically.

Even though this is only one paragraph, it is a long explanation for something that could be shorter. This paragraph took up 747 characters—14% of the AMCAS character limit and almost 17% of the AACOMAS limit. That is a lot. There is no need to mention the calculated GPAs. That is in the application. She tried to explain how grade replacement works to the Admissions Committee. She didn't need to do that.

So how do you make it shorter? Here is what we came up with:

As the eldest child of divorced parents, I became the caretaker to my disabled mother, which led to my decision to postpone my high school graduation and college matriculation.

This one sentence is now only 176 characters, more than 75% shorter than the previous example. It is short and to the point. The reader can infer from this sentence that there was a major life event that occurred around this student's senior year of high school. The reader then can look at her grades, if he or she wanted to, and see that there was some struggle around that time. The student still ended up with a good GPA, so focusing so much on it in the previous draft wasn't necessary. This student ended up with multiple acceptances to medical schools.

Another student who was accepted to medical school didn't mention in his personal statement that he was academically dismissed from his first college. He wrote about it in the secondary applications that asked about academic hardships.

Here is a further example of a student who decided to study nursing instead of her initial dream of becoming a physician:

As graduation neared, my dreams of applying to medical school were put on hold when my sister left her two small children in my care while she struggled to find work. My family was my priority, and I could not bear the thought of abandoning them in their time of need, even if it meant putting my future on hold. I decided to pursue a bachelor's degree of Nursing at State University so I could stay close to home. Nursing seemed like the most obvious career choice to get firsthand experience and patient interaction in the medical field. Shortly after starting the nursing program, my father was diagnosed with stage IV cancer. I was still helping my sister care for her children. With everything going on in my life, I buried my desire to become a doctor. I shifted my focus from medical school to starting my career as a nurse, so I would be able to help my family financially.

This is long, but it clearly lets the reader know why this student initially became a nurse and helps overcome any questions about her desires to become a physician. Some of the sentences and message can be tightened up to reduce the character count. This explanation does *show* a tremendous amount of selflessness to put her family ahead of her own desires—a great trait for physicians.

Here is one more example of a student writing about her struggles:

I dreamed about going to medical school, but I understood it was just that. A dream. My transition to adulthood was challenging in unique ways. I left home as soon as I could because I was expected to maintain the same level of responsibility that had so handicapped me in high school. I had saved thousands in a college fund, but my mother spent it. I had bad credit because she had used my identity. My father was well-off, but refused to help me. I worked several jobs at a time to support myself and my education. The difficulty of these years are reflected in my early transcripts.

In this example, the student refers to the financial struggles she had, which seemed to be caused by her parents. I don't like the way she started it though. If you want to be a physician, it's not a dream: it's a goal. No matter what obstacles you have to overcome, if you know you are meant to be a physician, then work towards that. The opening sentence is defeatist and doesn't give me confidence that she is going to work to survive medical school and residency. With that said, she is obviously applying to medical school now, so something has changed, and that's what the next part of her personal statement explores. Read her final draft, AR Final Draft, in full in Section II of this book.

As I mentioned earlier, not everything that you consider a red flag is one. Look at this example from a student who thought it would be a good idea to write about her MCAT struggles:

Persistence and "grit" became a common theme in my quest to become a doctor. So much so that I began to acclimate to the bumpy ride and just buckle up. The largest hurdle I experienced was my first attempt at the MCAT. After receiving my first score I was faced with the possibility that my greatest dream may not become a reality. An advisor told me that I was at the end of my road. The thought of losing my dream felt like losing a limb. I knew that becoming a doctor is more than a dream to me, it is part of who I am. I rejected the notion that I was at the end of my road in pursuing my passion of becoming a doctor. I was determined to fully engage myself to retake the MCAT and achieve my dreams.

You can see in this example that the student is determined to be a physician, and that's great, but needing to retake the MCAT isn't that high of a hurdle in the grand scheme of things. She took up 13% of her AMCAS essay and almost 16% of her AACOMAS essay with a red flag she didn't need to include. You may say that she included this story to show she's determined to get to medical school. You could make that argument, but I would point out that there are better ways to show **persistence and grit** in a personal statement. I would also argue that, to get to this stage in the process, every student has displayed some **persistence and grit**. Read her final draft, TJ Final Draft, in full in Section II of this book.

Traumatic Events

We have received many emails from students who have unfortunately been sexually assaulted at some point in their life. This traumatic event has been a spark for many to pursue becoming a physician. They ask me if they should discuss this in their personal statement.

Rape is a difficult topic for anyone to talk about. While it takes a lot of bravery to write about such a traumatic experience, and it may truly have inspired you to become a physician, you also don't want to make the reader uncomfortable as he or she is reading your personal statement. The reason is that you don't want the reader to only remember you because of their discomfort in reading your personal statement. There are ways to mention that you were attacked or assaulted without going in-depth into the details.

A student I worked with wrote this in her personal statement:

Intrigued by the field of medicine, I started my college career as a premed student. Things took a turn, however, when I was assaulted towards the end of my freshman year. I had been volunteering in a hospital, tutoring kids in math and science, and enjoying my college experience up to this point. I tried to continue on, but after a while realized I needed to take some time away from the campus to process the experience and to heal.

This paragraph helps explain a gap in her education without going into detail. Any logical person reading this personal statement will infer that she was raped, and it's much easier to digest this than going into deeply personal details. During a couple of her interviews, she was asked directly about this event and its impact.

If you've had a traumatic event in your life, and you feel it needs to be in your personal statement, then do it. Remember, your personal statement is meant to be personal. I don't want you to change your story just to avoid a particular topic.

What I'm trying to explain here is that you should tell your story in as few details as possible, leaving room for the rest of your journey, and making sure to keep the reader comfortable. The last thing you want is for the reader to put down your essay because they can't get through it. Save those deeper discussions for the interview.

Disability

I had a great conversation with Jeff, a legally blind physician, in Session 194 of *The Premed Years*[2]. The first time Jeff applied, he wrote extensively about his disability. It was all over his application. He still received several interviews and was even interviewed by an Ophthalmologist who tested his vision. I'm not a lawyer, but I think that is illegal. Jeff wasn't accepted anywhere after his first application cycle.

The second time Jeff applied, he took the advice of several advisors who told him not to mention his disability. He interviewed again, and this time was accepted. After his acceptance, he notified the school about his disability, and they accommodated him with no issues. Whether or not his disability played a role in his initial rejection is only known to the Admissions Committees that rejected him, but it was one more detail that could easily land him in the "no" pile.

Getting accepted to medical school is hard. As I'm writing this, the average acceptance rate is below 40%[3]. You should not give the Admissions Committee any easy reason to remove your application from contention because you want to write about a disability and spin it as a strength. The truth is, medical schools will have to accommodate you, and they may not want to. It's a sad reality. They can reject you, and you'll never know why.

[2] https://medicalschoolhq.net/194
[3] https://www.aamc.org/download/321494/data/factstablea16.pdf

Whether it's a physical disability or a mental health condition, I recommend you don't mention this in your personal statement. Get invited for the interview, and if they can see your disability when you're there, you can answer any questions about it then. Taking this approach, you will have the ability to make a great first impression so that they can see you for you and not your disability.

David, in Session 252 of *The Premed Years*[4], spoke openly about his ADHD and PTSD diagnoses. He wrote about his decision to only refer to his ADHD in his personal statement because it was an integral part of him deciding to become a physician.

The last thing I want you to do is to change your story to avoid writing about a disability. You need to be true to yourself and honest about your journey. If you make something up for your personal statement, and you're asked about it during an interview, it's usually pretty easy for the interviewer to see through your claims.

If a potential red flag defines your path, talk with your advisor about how to best tell that story without giving the Admissions Committee an easy way to reject your application.

Addiction

Drug and alcohol addiction is a catalyst for many to find meaning in their life. But as with a disability, you need to consider if this is something you want to advertise to the Admissions Committee as they are reviewing your application. If you've been sober for five years, does that give the Admissions Committee enough reassurance that once you encounter the rigors of medical school, you won't relapse?

If you've been lucky enough to not face any legal troubles from your addiction, and your journey is otherwise normal, I would completely avoid writing about your addiction. I always bring it back to the question—"Why would an Admissions Committee take a risk on you?" There are too many great applicants, and a big red flag, like addiction, can quickly land you in the "no" pile.

[4] https://medicalschoolhq.net/252

If you've had other red flags stemming from your addiction, like poor grades, arrests, or something else, then explain those things as best you can without going into too much detail about your addiction.

One student I recently did a mock interview with wrote about his addiction in his personal statement. The personal statement started with a story about his friend who overdosed on heroin. As the reader, I assumed that the student was addicted to heroin as well. It came out after the interview that he was actually addicted to Adderall instead. There is a huge difference in the stigma between those two drugs, and I recommended he contact the schools to let them know that, and that he was off the medication while earning great grades during the last several years of his schooling.

This is how the student wrote about his addiction:

The next five years were a rollercoaster ride through the world of addiction, taking a toll on my academic focus and motivation. Had I began my college career with the mindset I found in sobriety, I may have graduated with close to a 4.0. However, I wouldn't change the D in Calculus II, past mistakes, or all of the classes I withdrew from even if it were possible. Every moment of my struggle with addiction taught me lessons that I don't believe can be found in any textbook. I have experienced what it feels like to fail, to persevere, and above all I learned to appreciate and value my education.

You can read his full personal statement, CB Final Draft, by downloading free, extra essays at personalstatementbook.com/bonusessays.

Summary

The takeaway from this chapter is that you need to be true to who you are; tell your story. With that said, you also don't want to scare off the reader. With thousands of applications and interview invites only going to 10-20% of applicants, don't give them an obvious reason not to consider you as a student.

The goal of the application is to get the interview. During the interview, you'll have the opportunity to explore your story with the interviewers. In an interview, they'll have the ability to ask follow-up questions, making it a safer place to go deeper into something you truly feel needs to be mentioned.

CHAPTER EIGHT

SHOW DON'T TELL

When I'm editing personal statements one of the most common comments I type is "this is a TELLING statement, you need to SHOW me." Before we take a look at some examples, let's talk about why it's important to *show* and not *tell*. The advice to *show, not tell* is probably one of the most common pieces of advice given to all writers. It even has its own Wikipedia page[5].

When you *tell* the Admissions Committee, you are stating facts. You are describing what you have done and who you are to them. When you do this, you are writing like the majority of other applicants. This gets very boring for readers. This type of writing isn't memorable.

Your *telling* statements are going to convey very similar ideas to what other students are trying to convey. We discussed in the last chapter about how your experiences are going to be similar to thousands of other students; it's going to be the self-reflection that you have that will allow you to enhance each story and *show* the Admissions Committee why you chose to tell that story.

[5] https://en.wikipedia.org/wiki/Show,_don't_tell

Showing, on the other hand, is very memorable. As I'm writing this, I can easily recall some great stories that students wrote in their personal statements that I have read over the years. They did such a great job *showing* me what they were trying to convey that I felt like I was there with them.

Humans have five senses: sight, hearing, touch, smell, and taste. When you *show* in your personal statement, you are helping elicit these senses in the reader. The more senses you can activate, the more memorable your story will be. Have you ever been drawn back to a memory based on a sound or smell? This is exactly what you want for your reader.

The most memorable personal statements that I have read didn't just *tell* me that the student volunteered and had a great time; they *showed* me what they did, the impact that they had on an individual, or the impact that the experience had on them. They *showed* me by painting a picture and using words that made me feel like I was there; words that activated my senses.

Let's take a look at some *telling* statements and see how we can improve them.

One student opened up her personal statement like this:

Even as a child I have always been fairly shy. Whether I am meeting new people, starting a new job, or even at family parties I tend to be quiet and reserved and have thus found myself in supportive roles. I have worked in sales support the majority of my time at Super Store and have noticed I enjoy family parties most when I am helping to cook, clean, and be of service. I had feared that this may be an obstacle to thriving as a physician, but I soon learned that it is a blessing rather than an obstacle. Volunteering at the Community Clinic for the uninsured in St. Louis provided my first true one-on-one experience with patients. When performing intakes of new patients or seeing return patients to present to the clinician, I was at their service. This was when I found my quiet nature to be a benefit instead of a hindrance; I was there to listen, take notes, and ask questions.

Let's break down some of these sentences and see how they are *telling* the reader what is happening:

"Even as a child I have always been fairly shy." This is the first sentence of the personal statement. The first sentence is *telling* the reader what could be a potentially negative trait about the student. I would tell the student to remove it.

"…I tend to be quiet and reserved and have thus found myself in supportive roles." Here again, the student is continuing down the path of *telling* the reader about this struggle. Being a physician involves connecting with patients and families and interacting with the healthcare team. You can see that, as she finishes the paragraph, she is trying to *sell* her shyness as a positive trait, which doesn't come off well.

"When performing intakes of new patients or seeing return patients to present to the clinician, I was at their service." "I was at their service" is *telling* the reader what the student did. This could have been much stronger if the student had *showed* the reader an encounter with one of the patients. I'll give an example of this next.

"This was when I found my quiet nature to be a benefit instead of a hindrance; I was there to listen, take notes, and ask questions." The closing takeaway is the sales pitch to the reader—I'm quiet, and reserved, but *I* think that I will make a good physician because of it. *Telling* the reader that you will be a good physician is not the role of the personal statement.

Because the whole paragraph is a pitch to the reader about the student's shyness and how it will help her be a physician, I would have told her to delete the whole thing. Let's take a look, though, at how we can change the section about the interaction with the patients at the clinic.

Here is how it can be written to *show* the reader her service:

I led Jane back to the exam room where the physician would see her after I was done checking her in. This was her first visit and I could tell by the tone in her voice that she was nervous. As I do with every patient, I asked her how we could help her today. As she began talking, I listened and made sure that she knew I was paying attention, even as I was taking notes. The longer we talked, the more I could see Jane relax…

Can you see how this partial paragraph is *showing* the reader how the student was being of service and not just *telling* the reader that she is. The action words of "led," "talking," and "listening" are all engaging the reader's senses. Writing about the "tone in her voice" forces the reader to imagine what it might sound like. This is how you want your personal statement to read—showing the reader *what* you are doing instead of just *telling* it to him or her.

One of the quickest ways to determine if your personal statement is too much of a *telling* personal statement, and not *showing*, is to count the number of times you use "I [verb]" statements: "I watched," "I shadowed," "I began." The more of these types of sentences you have, the more I know your personal statement will be *telling* and not *showing*.

If you are constantly stating, "I joined," "I led," or any other statement, this should give you a sense that you are not headed in the right direction. This does not mean your stories are wrong. It just means that the *way* you are writing about them could be more effective.

Don't worry if you have "I [verb]" statements. There is no way to remove them completely from your writing. Just make sure that they are used sparingly and see if you can reword the sentence to something more *showing*.

Here is another example from a student recalling the moment he realized that he needed to become a physician:

Call it an epiphany but right at that moment I knew I had come full circle. I had an overwhelming sense of illumination in my heart and soul. That moment I began formulating a game plan to achieve my passion and my calling which had never left my heart: that of being a physician.

Here, he *told* me that this was his passion and calling, but he never went on to explain **why** it was. He continued to write about what happened next. Despite being a more *telling* personal statement, this student was interviewed and accepted to medical school. Read his final draft, JR Final Draft, in full in Section II of this book.

Here's another example of telling:

In 2013, I had already begun my journey to change my life and career to one of service to others. It was during this time that I watched the catastrophic results of the explosion. I found myself feeling humble, yet hopeful with the anticipation that in a few years, I would be running toward the scene to be of service to those in need, rather than simply sitting idly by watching the news, feeling helpless.

After helping the student change his words to *show* me, this is what he came up with:

Watching the smoke rising from the catastrophic explosion, I felt helpless. I was sitting watching on the news, when what I really wanted to be doing was running toward the scene to help those in need. I knew at this moment that I had made the right decision three years ago to begin on my path to medical school.

It's shorter and more impactful. It's more memorable. With more active words like "watching" instead of "watched," the student paints a picture of him sitting and being part of this tragedy. It pulls the reader in and forces them to be there with the student. When you help the reader activate their different senses, you're helping them make your personal statement leave a stronger impression. Read his final draft, JD Final Draft, in full in Section II of this book.

More Examples

Here are some great examples of students going from *telling* to *showing*. This is an early draft from one student writing about acting:

After graduating from State University, I spent several years working as an actress. A genuine curiosity about the human psyche is what drew me to the acting profession.

This is a very *telling* statement. It's not engaging any senses; it's just stating the facts.

Compare that with this final draft version *showing* me:

I stood up from my desk and tried again, repeating the lines that were burned into my brain from hours of repetition and rehearsal. I imagined the hunger pangs that pierced my abdomen, the dull headache, the weakness in my limbs, and the utter exhaustion of my spirit. I was long past the memorization stage and now onto discovering how to make the playwright's words come alive. I had to discover how to infuse my performance with the physicality brought about by chronic starvation and the mental anguish from being imprisoned without an end in sight. I was fortunate enough to have the lead role, Fania Fenelon, in the production of Playing for Time by Arthur Miller. The play was based on the true story of Fania, a French singer using her musical talent to survive Auschwitz during WWII. It was my job to bring her truth to my performance and honor her story.

I'm immediately picturing this student as she is rehearsing her lines. I'm drawn into what she is doing and thinking and wondering why. I'm intrigued and want to know more. This is great *showing*. Read her final draft, JW Final Draft, in full in Section II of this book.

Here's a student who opened one of his drafts *telling* the reader about early interests and struggle:

Over the years, my medical interests helped me excel in the science track in high school to the point of becoming a certified first aid and CPR instructor. I knew that I wanted to be a physician. However, after high school, the stark reality of my family's humble status came to bear. I was compelled to find a job to support my family financially, tempering any hopes of going to college, or becoming a physician. However, with great determination, I was able to secure a one-year partial tuition scholarship, and in total opposition to my parents' wishes, I went to college.

Compare that to this opening, where he paints a great picture for me, helping engage my senses with his descriptions of the surroundings and his environment:

We stood outside, a mass of bodies sweating in the sweltering Florida sunshine. Around us were the gritty, low-income apartments and run-down single family homes that bracketed the parking lot where we gathered. The main door was decorated with a velveteen congratulatory red ribbon that signified the Chamber of Commerce was about to perform another ribbon cutting ceremony for a new business. This was our business, One Health, a free clinic in Tampa, FL.

This isn't creative writing. This is a great paragraph that shows me who this student is—a business owner; it immediately piques my interest and makes me want to keep reading. That is the first goal of each sentence—to make the reader want to keep reading. Read his final draft, JuD Final Draft, in full in Section II of this book.

Here's one from a draft of a nontrad:

There were fourteen beady-eyes staring up at me. Seven first graders were eagerly awaiting to begin their first music lesson of the year. Unbeknownst to them, I was frozen in place filled to the brim with dread while my mind was ruminating on my huge mistake of a career choice. My lifelong dream of becoming a music educator quickly soured.

The descriptive words and phrases "beady-eyes," "eagerly awaiting, "frozen in place," and "ruminating" all draw the reader in. This student did a great job of *showing* the reader that she was a first-grade teacher and had an epiphany that she didn't want to be one anymore.

She could have easily *told* the reader the same thing by saying, "I was a first-grade music teacher and I realized that what had been my lifelong dream of being a music educator wasn't what I wanted to do anymore."

Read this next example and tell me if your heart starts racing a little bit:

Sprinting from a beating helicopter and fighting to see through the dust and night vision goggles in the middle of the night in Iraq, I was doing everything I could to clear a safe path for my strike force. Trying to see through the grit was like trying to blink away sweat while opening the door to a hot oven. I had to push the pace; speed and surprise were our best security in raids like these. I didn't feel like a "barrelchested freedom fighter"; I initially felt like an impostor. I was an Army special operations explosive ordnance disposal team leader, and I was absolutely terrified. What was I doing here? How did I find myself in this position, responsible for this many lives? I was as scared as I have ever been. Along with 60 strangers that I had met only hours before, we made it through the region of the world most densely laden with improvised explosive devices that night; it was the first of many.

Do you want to keep reading to see what he has to say next? I certainly do. This is the perfect example of a student highlighting who he is through storytelling, by *showing* the reader his path. Read his final draft, DB Final Draft, in full in Section II of this book.

Summary

If you don't take anything else from this book, you should be left with the messages in this chapter. Review your writing and look for those "I [verb]" statements. The more of those you have, the more *telling* that you are likely doing. That doesn't mean you can avoid them all together. The last example of the student running from the helicopter had "I [verb]" statements, but they were in the context of his story.

Have someone take a look at your personal statement and ask them if they were intrigued by your story, or if they just felt like you were telling them about who you are. Ask them if there were any parts that didn't activate their senses or that didn't make them want to find out more about you. If you can improve and refine those sections, you're on your way to writing a great personal statement.

In the end, you'll find the right balance for you and your writing style. There is no perfect ratio of *telling* vs. *showing*. Just remember that *showing* is much more memorable, which is what you want.

CHAPTER NINE

HOW TO BE UNIQUE AND NOT CLICHÉD

By the time a reader is done reading a good personal statement, it will have told them precisely what your inspiration was—what exactly planted that seed of being a physician in your head. The most common topics of personal statements are personal illnesses or injuries, family illnesses, injuries, or deaths, family members who are physicians or other healthcare providers, wanting to do more in a situation, and having a pure fascination with science among others.

Here are a few examples of students writing about their initial experiences:

Despite the wonderful experiences I had while acting, I did not feel fulfilled. I realized that I longed for a career in which I could have a direct impact on people's lives. After watching Dr. H fight for my father's quality of life, I began to realize that a career in medicine might be a perfect fit for me.

This student was a former actress who turned premed following her exposure to medicine during a family member's illness. Read her final draft, JW Final Draft, in full in Section II of this book.

It never crossed my mind that someone could come out into that hallway and see someone else lying helpless, perhaps dying, on the floor and not immediately take action. Her words had two profound effects on me. First, they made me reflect on why I was compelled to act at the site of a fellow human being in need. I possessed innate tendencies to help my fellow man. This also explained why I felt such a strong pull to leave my successful career and pursue the path of a physician.

This student reacted to a situation in a way that others didn't, but couldn't help as much as he wanted because he didn't know how. Read his final draft, KL Final Draft, in full in Section II of this book.

I have always had a fascination for human physiology due to the numerous visits I paid to emergency rooms as a child for injuries sustained while playing. While still in high school, I discovered the opportunity to receive a certification as a nurse assistant and sought after it knowing it would place me in an experienced position as my college years neared. I credit this education as a catalyst for pursuing medicine.

This student had personal injuries that led to an interest in science, pushing her down a path to obtain more and more exposure. Read her final draft, SC Final Draft, in full in Section II of this book.

You may be thinking that these are all very clichéd reasons to enter medicine. Using the strictest definition of cliché, you might be right. But the general definition[6] is a *"phrase or opinion that is overused and betrays a lack of original thought."* The reasons listed in the above stories are not phrases or opinions as the definition lays out. Rather, they are original thoughts because they are personal experiences. Experiences are **always** original.

[6] https://en.oxforddictionaries.com/definition/cliche

I can give every student the same book to read and then give them a survey, asking him or her what lessons they learned. I can ask about what he or she liked the most or didn't like. Every student will read that book through the lens of his or her life and see and learn something completely different from the next student.

Your parent getting sick and motivating you to become a physician is different from my experiences with my dad being sick my whole life from type 1 diabetes. My experience is different from anyone else's experience because I felt and experienced and formed memories based on everything else that had happened in my life to that point. **No one else** has had those same experiences.

Think about all of the sons and daughters of parents who are sick or die. Only a small fraction of those children are now pursuing medicine because of those experiences. It's not the experience itself that draws them to medicine—it's the totality of their experiences combined with the experience of their parents being ill that has propelled them along this path.

Being Unique

Now that you hopefully understand that it's hard to be clichéd if you're writing about your experiences, the question is, how do you identify the right experiences out of all of those you've had and fit those stories into 4,500-5,300 characters?

You need to edit your life experiences and cut out the stuff that doesn't tell the reader *exactly* why you want to be a physician or *exactly* what you've experienced to help you make that decision. Does that mean that you write about every patient interaction? Not at all. It means you figure out the **one** experience that has left a significant enough impact on you that you can *show* the reader through your words how that situation strengthened your desire to become a physician. Ask yourself, "Why was this moment so memorable for me?" When you reflect, you can then describe.

The first time you interacted with a physician may have been during a personal or family health issue. Students tend to shy away from this as their initial interest in medicine because they don't feel it's unique enough. They try to be too creative, and when they do that, the reader is typically left confused about your true motivation. If the reader is confused, or if they still don't understand why you are applying to medical school, your application is going to end up in the "do not interview" pile.

The problem with thinking that your story isn't unique is that this might influence you into changing who you are and what your initial motivations were to pursue this path. Doing so completely ignores the **personal** part of the personal statement.

Here's the interesting thing about being unique. If you are writing about *your* experience, it is 100% unique. Have you ever watched a movie with a friend and, afterward, you both have completely different thoughts about it? Everything that you have gone through in your life is unique to you. The way you were raised, the neighborhood you grew up in, the schools that you attended, all give you unique lenses through which to look.

Take a look at what this student learned from his early years:

I can't stop staring at the door. Doors have become a recurring theme in my life, and this clinic was just another in a series of entrances to opportunities that have shaped my life. Immediately, my mind was seamlessly transported to the humid living room of my parents' small home. I stared at the forbidden door that held the mysteries of childbirth behind it. I heard my mother, a seasoned midwife, utter clipped instructions to laboring mothers. Once in a while, I peeked from behind the forbidden doors and beheld the importance of my mother's work in communities that lacked resources and access, where she provided midwifery services to mothers who otherwise could not afford it. These moments in my formative years impressed upon me the importance of being a medical provider in communities such as ours.

While you are reading that story, you can't help but put yourself in this student's shoes. You are immediately transported in your mind to a living room, peeking out from behind a door. This student did an amazing job of **showing** us his earliest memories of service to the community in a medical sense. This specific student is the only one who can tell this story. It's unique. If he had just stated that he volunteered in an underserved clinic and wants to give back to others who are underserved, I could copy and paste this into another application and not notice any difference. This kind of interchangeability is something you want to avoid.

I can't stress it enough—the personal statement is there to tell the reader why *you* want to be a doctor. What is *your* why? What are *your* experiences that have led you down this path? That is really all it should do. Unfortunately, many students miss this simple point and try to be too fancy. Fortunately for you, you are reading this book and won't make that mistake.

Knowing that your experiences are unique to you, it's okay to write about personal health issues as the initial "a-ha" moment. It's okay to write about the illness of a family member as your *initial* exposure to healthcare. It's okay to write about how those experiences were the launching point of your motivations regarding becoming a physician. It's not a cliché. It's your story. What you can't do is just stop there. That's just the *initial* exposure.

As I've mentioned previously, I like to use the analogy of growing a plant. Your initial exposure is the planting of the seed. What was that initial experience that planted the seed for you? When I have discussions with students about starting their personal statements and what to write about, I'll ask about their initial motivations. A lot of times they shy away from some of what they presume to be more clichéd responses.

One student I recently worked with talked about working as an EMT as his initial interest. When I discussed this with him, it didn't seem like he had much to say. He wasn't passionate talking about it. It also didn't explain why he became an EMT in the first place—how did he end up in healthcare if he is saying being an EMT was his interest? You can't already be in healthcare and say that is what interested you to pursue it. Why did he become an EMT to begin with? Why is he pursuing becoming a physician now? When we drilled down further, we discovered that his initial interest in medicine came from a sports injury, which is common for many students. He was hesitant to write about it because he thought it wouldn't sound unique. I quickly put that argument to rest. It was his injury, playing his sport, causing him a crisis that ultimately led him to where he was now, an EMT. The experience he had as an EMT motivated him to explore being a physician even further. It is stories like this that give the reader a lot of valuable information about your journey and your goals. In fact, this student's journey was very similar to mine.

I hurt my shoulder playing baseball. I went to an Orthopedic Surgeon, then to an athletic trainer and physical therapist. I thought I was going to be a physical therapist because I wanted to help other people rehab to get back to their sports. It wasn't until I dissected a cat in anatomy in high school that I decided that I wanted to cut people open for a living. I married the two passions of sports and surgery and decided that Orthopedic Surgery was the specialty that I wanted to pursue.

Ultimately, that's not what ended up happening, but that was my initial desire and something that I've written about in my personal statements and in other essays about my journey. You can't fake who you are. You can't pretend that the initial experiences that have opened your eyes up to medicine aren't there. You can't make up stories to tell yourself to seem 'unique.' You need to be you. This is a personal statement. It is all about you. It doesn't matter if half of the other students are all writing about injuries that have led them to this journey; if that is what led you down this journey too, write about it.

Storytelling

I explained earlier about the Hero's Journey. This is where you separate yourself from other students. Just because Luke Skywalker from *Star Wars* and Neo from *The Matrix* are characters who follow the Hero's Journey, doesn't mean their stories are the same. Each writer has *shown* the reader or audience member different pieces of each character's journey through storytelling.

We see Luke as a child, being called to action as his aunt and uncle are killed and his journey to becoming a Jedi after meeting Obi-Wan and Yoda. Through George Lucas' storytelling, Luke Skywalker becomes a character for which you root.

Even though Neo's story follows a similar hero archetype, The Wachowskis' storytelling is different. Neo is a completely different character because of his background and experiences.

Showing the reader your journey through storytelling is how you stand out and avoid being clichéd. The worst personal statements are the ones that just *tell* me that they were sick, they loved their doctor, and then they shadowed and knew they wanted to be a doctor. The best ones *show* me who they are and what experiences they've had.

Check out this great example of *showing* the reader your experiences:

"You should go talk to M. She was an actress, just like you!" Per the charge nurse's instructions, I knocked on M's door. I introduced myself as a volunteer and asked if she would be willing to participate in a patient feedback survey. She paused and then burst into tears. I stood in the doorway and said, "I'm not just here for the survey. I can also listen if you need someone to talk to." M told me that none of her friends had come to visit, she just found out she had cancer, and an hour ago she received an IRS notice which would bankrupt her. Her world was crumbling around her and she did not see a point in continuing on. I did not say much; I held her hand and listened.

This student could have easily said that she volunteered in the hospital and *told* me that she walked around to see different patients and do patient feedback surveys. That is how most students write their personal statements.

This example, though, is so much more powerful. It *shows* me something about the student. It *shows* me that she is empathetic, and a good listener. It *shows* me what she was doing. She didn't have to *tell* me any of it. The student finished the paragraph a little later with her *why*. Read her final draft, JW Final Draft, in full in Section II of this book.

Summary

If the core of your personal statement is about your own experiences, then you are not being clichéd. Write about your experiences, your emotions, and the impacts each experience had on you.

Write your personal statement based on what has motivated you to become a physician, not anything else. Don't worry about what you think the Admissions Committee *wants to read*. If you try to do this, you'll stumble into the cliché because your thoughts will no longer be original. Next, we'll cover what to avoid in your personal statement.

CHAPTER TEN

WHAT TO AVOID IN YOUR PERSONAL STATEMENT

I hope that at this point in the book, you understand how important it is to write about why you want to be a doctor. If you are trying to do something else with your personal statement, then that is the first thing I will tell you not to write about.

If you think that telling the reader some random story from your past is going to separate you from the other students—that it's going to make your application stand out—I'll tell you to avoid writing about that. When you bring these types of stories into your personal statement, you're now writing an argumentative paper on why you think you're better, or why you think you will be a great student. The goal of the personal statement is to show me **why you want to be a physician.**

There are several other things that students often don't consider as well.

Lying and Exaggerating

I feel weird even putting this one in the book, but here I am. There are students who, every year, try to pull a fast one and exaggerate something about themselves in their personal statement or in their application. Don't do this.

If you have a committee letter from your undergrad, and they want to see your application before they write your letter—and they know you're exaggerating, or aren't being truthful—**they will** call you out in your committee letter.

Even if you don't have a committee letter, don't do this. The last thing you want to do is get caught in a lie. You'll ruin your chances of acceptance to *any* medical school.

Emotional topics

If you cry when talking about certain topics, maybe the passing of a parent, or another emotional subject, don't write about it. You may think that since it's written, it's safe to do because the Admissions Committee member isn't watching you write your personal statement. While it's true that you can cry all you want when writing your personal statement, what you don't want to happen is the interviewer asking you about the events that you wrote about, which will bring up those emotions during the interview.

People cry, that's okay, but in a professional setting, with an interviewer trying to determine if she wants you to take care of her mom, you want to avoid it. If you start bawling in the interview, she is going to picture you bawling when you're giving bad news to her mom.

So even if you think it's safe to **write** about emotional subjects, understand that they will be fair game when it comes to the interview. If you don't think you can maintain your composure when discussing this part of your life in an interview, don't write about it in your personal statement.

Doctor or Medical Student Skills

The personal statement is not the place to tell the reader that you think you have the skills and traits necessary to be a physician. It's not the time to show that you *think* you'll be a great physician in the future.

I once got an email from a student I was helping. He wrote this:

I want the medical schools to know how much I want this, and I want them to know that I hope to be a great physician in the future.

This is a very common trap all the way along the application process. Students think that by writing about how much they *really* want this, that they can do it, that they are dedicated to it, then the Admissions Committee is going to say, "Hey, look, we finally found one who knows that this is what they want!"

I would hope that **every** student applying to medical school is dedicated to this process. It's nearly impossible to get through the premed classes, take the MCAT, and apply to medical school without being dedicated. Yes, there are going to be a few who slip through the cracks and are only doing this because their parents want them to do it. There are even the ones who think that the physician *lifestyle* is what they want, and not necessarily *being* a physician.

However, your job is not to write about yourself with the aim of highlighting your strengths. Too many students like to describe their dedication, compassion, intelligence, teamwork, and other skills. Again, this is just what the *student thinks* the reader wants to read about. You will **not** be invited for an interview based on such statements.

You will be invited for an interview because you are interesting, not because you tell the reader you will be a great physician.

Here is an example of a nontraditional student selling her skills she learned as a massage therapist:

I have developed and honed interpersonal, team, and practical skills that will be invaluable as a physician, such as: taking health histories, asking keen questions, balancing compassionate care with efficiency, an understanding of referral relationships, knowledge of integrative healing modalities, and solid communication skills.

As soon as you start writing your personal statement in a way that tries to sell yourself to the Admissions Committee member, you are no longer writing a personal statement. Instead, you are writing a persuasive paper about why they should interview you. If your paper ends up doing that, then you've failed.

Let your stories and your path show the reader how interesting you are and let them determine if your experiences match up to the types of students for which they are looking.

Consider how this nontraditional student tried to sell the reader her skills acquired by being a mom:

> *Like a doctor, a mother works long hours, is always on call and must carefully observe her charges to determine what is amiss when they are unable to communicate. A mother must constantly learn new things as her children are everchanging, and she must judiciously seek out evidence-based advice in a world full of opinions. When faced with a difficult task, I tell myself, if I have raised 5 kids, I can do anything.*

This is almost 10% of an AACOMAS application essay and none of this needed to be included. Knowing that a student is a mother tells me all of this already.

You have to remember that medical schools are trying to build communities with each class. In that community, they want students who will contribute their unique backgrounds and personalities. They can only do that if you are honest about who you are in your personal statement and discuss your journey authentically. Make their jobs easier by staying away from trying to sell yourself.

Here is a good example of what could have been a powerful story about helping a patient but turned out to be something else entirely:

> *One day, while on call, an elderly patient had slipped and fallen on the ground. Treating for a spinal injury, the other EMTs and I, worked together to attach a cervical collar and backboard the patient onto a stretcher. Working as a unit, we delegated roles: I was in charge of stabilizing the head, two other EMTs were in charge of logrolling the patient, and the fourth had to slide the backboard under. To prevent any miscalculated actions that could prove detrimental to the patient, I told my team to "log roll on three," and proceeded to count to three. In such an experience, I learned that by coordinating our actions, we can move towards treating the patient more*

efficiently and effectively. The skills I gained as an EMT to function in a team successfully will be an asset for my future colleagues and patients.

Did you take away the same message that I did? I took away that the student wanted me to know that she has good communication and teamwork skills and that she thinks those will help her in the future.

The goal is not to tell me **why** you think you're going to be a good physician. It's to tell me **why you want to be one**. This story could have been much stronger if she told me about the patient. How was she able to help the patient? Why did that make her feel good? Why does she want more of that in the future?

She did a much better job later in her personal statement when she told another story of a patient encounter:

I quickly administered him an EpiPen, and then sat with him to monitor his vitals. After he normalized, he gave me a hug and said "thank you, you saved my life." It was at this moment that I felt an overwhelming sense of gratification and happiness. This camp was a second home for me, and for me to be able to use my knowledge to save those that I considered family was heartwarming and reassuring of the path I was following. Treating the child made me eager to expand my knowledge of medicine and determine to become a physician so that I could provide care to a broader community.

With this story, I'm able to picture her taking care of the patient and imagine the patient's response to her. I'm able to see why it was so important to her that she mentioned it in her personal statement.

Knowing the Life or Struggles of Physicians

Another twist on this same trend is when students try to comment on what being a physician is like. While you may have had some experience shadowing and getting clinical experience, you are not a physician. Yet.

Some readers won't care. Some may take offense to you claiming you understand the life of a physician. I've seen students write about understanding the difficulties they are going to face, the type of person a physician has to be, and so on.

Here is a good example from a personal statement:

Being a physician is one of the most important teaching positions of all.

This is a very benign comment, but when a student claims to know different aspects of being a physician, it can come across badly. I usually tell students to avoid these types of statements.

Nontraditional students fall into this trap very easily because they usually have great experiences outside of school and try to include these in their personal statement. This fails the first rule of the personal statement: it needs to be personal. As soon as you start forcing in information that you think will be relevant for the reader to know, especially regarding skills and traits, it's no longer personal. (The one exception to this is any red flags which may need to be discussed.)

Here is a great example of someone who is changing professions after a long career in the computer programming industry. This is from his first application attempt, prior to working with me. Read his final draft, JD Final Draft, in full in Section II of this book.

My career as a programmer and computer engineer has helped prepare me for medical school in many ways. It has given me many years of experience in honing my analytical skills. In my job, I have regularly been tasked with determining the source of issues with only an array of symptoms, a number of tests that can be run, and my own deductive abilities. By running both invasive and non-invasive tests on my system, I could eliminate possibilities until I had identified the cause of software issues. While working in the data storage industry, I have been trained to treat failure as an unacceptable outcome. It is vital to maintain data integrity in the customer market. There is a high degree of sensitivity to issues that could compromise integrity. As important as this is and although it has synergy with medical care, it admittedly pales in comparison to care of human life. With medical training, my proven analytical skills can work together to assist in determining health issues of patients.

The student is trying really hard, and taking up **a lot** of space (20% of his TMDSAS essay), to compare his prior career to medicine and show that he has the skills necessary to be a good medical student and physician. The job of the Admissions Committee is to look at your experiences and your essays and determine if *they* think that you have what it takes to be a valued member of the medical school. They will be trying to picture you as a caring and compassionate physician in the future, but it is not *your* job to tell them *you* think you have what it takes.

Avoid the Résumé

Your personal statement should not look like a résumé. Too many students just give an overview of their life. When you structure your personal statement in this way, the reader will likely get turned off and toss your application into the digital shredder, also known as the "do not interview" pile. These types of essays are not impactful. They are not memorable. This is the opposite effect that you want to have on the Admissions Committee.

When you follow a résumé type template, everything that you include in your personal statement will likely already be in your application. Your primary application should not be used as an outline for your personal statement. Why force the reader to sit through reading your story twice—once through with the formatted application and another time through with your personal statement?

When I'm giving feedback on personal statements, another very common phrase that I use is, "this is an extracurricular description."

Here is an example of a student going too far into writing about her experiences for a personal statement. None of these experiences are told in a way that helps the reader understand the student's motivations for becoming a physician.

In my undergraduate years, I was eager to find others who had similar dreams of becoming a doctor. I began volunteering in my community and joined several organizations to surround myself with those that shared my passion. I also found myself captivated by research conducted by one of my professors. At this point in my education I had taken several classes that explained the scientific method in detail, but it wasn't until I worked in Dr. Smith's lab that I was able to appreciate the scientific method and all of its beauty. In her lab, we worked to find the neural basis of addiction so that oneday pharmacological interventions could help combat the effects of alcohol withdrawal. It was fascinating to think that every medication being prescribed by physicians today started with the very steps we were taking. Long hours in the lab, reading, studying, and learning with the hope that these new findings would help improve the quality of someone's life inspired me. Every detail and every data entry was important; I was enamored by the power of research.

This student could easily have written about everything here in an extracurricular description.

Referencing the Application

Your personal statement needs to stand on its own. You should be able to take it out of your application and hand it to someone, and they should be able to understand **why** you want to be a physician.

The personal statement should not lean on the rest of the application to fill in gaps. Don't reference anything else from your application in your personal statement.

An example of this would be:

"As you can see from the extracurricular list, I've been very involved in research..."

Write your personal statement assuming that the Admissions Committee member will only have access to the statement and nothing else. This will help force you to look at it as though it's a separate document.

But My Extracurriculars are the Reason I Want to be a Physician!

I'm sure you're yelling right now, "I want to be a physician **because** of my extracurriculars, so how can I not write about them?!"

When I tell you not to write about your extracurriculars, I mean don't give me extra details about them. And definitely, don't list them. If there is a story that has reinforced your desire to be a physician, tell me that story.

Here is an example of what I mean:

Plan in place I returned to college spring 2012 and shortly after started working full-time as a phlebotomist at Norman Regional Hospital while going to school. One particular day stands out above all others.

The extra details regarding 2012, working full-time, and the hospital is taking up very valuable character space, and they just don't need to be there. The real heart of the message comes after the student makes the transition to the story. Read his final draft, JR Final Draft, in full in Section II of this book.

General Statements and Facts

"This is a very general statement" is one of the other more common pieces of feedback that I give to students. Almost all of the time, the statements students include are true, but are they really needed?

Remember, you only have 4,500-5,300 characters to fit in your story explaining why you want to be a doctor. Do you really want to waste any of that saying something that isn't true to who you are?

Let's look at this example:

Having to decide on a future career at a young age was a difficult choice for me to make. There was an entire world of careers, each different and unique, but which path was meant for me? This confusion made me feel as if I was stuck in a jungle and the only way out was that I had to explore my interests to open a path to my future. My interest in medicine first piqued when I took my first anatomy and physiology class in high school.

Is deciding on a career early hard? Of course it is. Is it unique to this applicant? Not at all. Is there an entire world of careers? Yep. Is the only way to figure it out by exploring interests? Definitely.

This example was the opening to a personal statement. These three very general statements hit me before they even got to the heart of the question, "Why medicine?" Read her final draft, VY Final Draft, in full in Section II of this book.

Students also like to write about their major, GPA, and MCAT scores.

Look how this student addressed a career change in her personal statement:

I needed to fully invest myself in medicine to be on the forefront of action, so I enrolled in a post-baccalaureate premed program at State University where I received a second Bachelor's in Health Sciences with a 3.85 GPA.

This information is in the application. It's not needed in a personal statement. It's not a statement that makes this student unique and it's not giving the committee any new information to help them make their decision. On top of that, it takes up almost 5% of the total characters for the osteopathic application essay.

Quotes

Go on any social media site, and you'll be sure to find a great quote image within the first couple of flicks of the finger. Quotes are great for motivating you during your frequent moments of procrastination on Instagram, but you probably shouldn't use them in your personal statement.

Quotes are other people's words, not yours. It's weird giving you this advice because as you'll read in my personal statement, I used a quote. I didn't have advice from others when I wrote my personal statement. I thought quotes were great. That's probably where you are coming from too.

Every character counts when it comes to your personal statement, and most students struggle to cut out sentences and dig through the thesaurus looking for shorter words that won't completely change their message.

If for some reason you just *have* to have a quote in your personal statement, keep it short and don't use it as a central focal point. Make sure to give the author of the quote credit too.

Themes

Earlier on in the book, I mentioned that the personal statement is not a creative writing piece. Some students walk the line and some even flat out cross into theming their whole essay.

When you theme your essay, you're just distracting the reader from your true message. I can't mention it enough, but every single character that doesn't need to be in your personal statement needs to be removed. It's just taking up space.

One personal statement I looked at had these theme references in it:

- *This confusion made me feel as if I was stuck in a jungle.*
- *Provided for me a path out of the jungle and into the world of medicine.*
- *I was slowly making my way out of the jungle.*
- *I noticed my peers changing their career paths and navigating through their own jungles.*
- *Escaping the jungle helped me find my way to medicine.*

Each one of these statements guides the reader through the student's journey of wanting to be a physician. When I'm reading a personal statement about why you want to be a doctor, the last thing that I expect to read about is the jungle. This is a great example of a student trying to get a little too fancy when writing their personal statement.

Here's another example of a theme being too much:

- *I am engaged. And like my friends who are engaged, but in a much different way, I am elated.*
- *Engaged is a word a woman of my age, from a small town in rural Alabama, hears quite often.*
- *I am fully and deeply engaged in a wholly different way.*
- *I learned at a young age to be fully engaged in every activity and be present in everything I did.*

The theme of being engaged continued on throughout the draft. Read her first draft, TJ First Draft, in full in Section II of this book.

Negativity

Negativity is a very quick application killer. If you're negative about your prior career, a past professor, or any other aspect of your life in your personal statement or anywhere else in your application, you are giving the Admissions Committee an easy reason to pass on inviting you for an interview.

The goal of the personal statement and the rest of your primary and secondary application is to have the Admission Committee interested in knowing who you are, that you are motivated to push through the tough times, and if you are going to be a good fit with the rest of the class. Any negativity in your application shows them that you likely aren't who they are looking for.

Here is one example of a student writing about her premed journey and some of her early struggles:

> *I grew bored memorizing facts and became more interested in assessing and solving problems.*

This immediately made me wonder if she was also going to grow bored during medical school. Guess what? Medical school involves a lot of memorizing too.

Another student described a patient as *ornery*. If you're already frustrated with "ornery" patients enough to mention it in your personal statement, an Admissions Committee isn't going to want to see how much more frustrated you're going to get during your training.

Bad Physician Encounters

Another common trap that students fall into is writing negatively about physicians as part of their motivation to become physicians themselves. A physician treating your family member poorly shouldn't be the main reason you want to be a physician. While it may have opened your eyes to the world of medicine, writing negatively about that physician won't accomplish anything.

Here is an example of a student discussing what happened to her mom:

> *After my mother was told that she would get better by attending psychological counseling, I was in disbelief. Her symptoms were real but this doctor thought she was imagining them. I could not fathom how a doctor could dismiss a patient instead of digging deeper into the matter, so I felt the absolute need to change this approach.*

How does she know that doctor dismissed the patient? As a human, I can understand how someone wouldn't want to hear that their symptoms might be psychological. As a physician, I have learned how powerful the brain can be at manifesting symptoms. If I read this in a personal statement, I would worry that the student's main motivation is to prove this doctor wrong.

Here's another example of a student discussing negative aspects of healthcare to the statement's detriment:

> *I have observed trembling hands of physicians in front of helpless patients being intubated or their frustrated eyes before administrative policies that hinder them from providing effective patient care.*

Abbreviations and Jargon

I was in the Air Force for five years of my life. I know a lot of abbreviations. The abbreviations that I know though may not be ones that you know. Did you know that OPSEC mean Operations Security? Back when I was still serving, it would be very easy for me to use this shorthand outside of the work environment, around my civilian friends. They wouldn't have understood what I was talking about. The same holds true for your personal statement.

If you've done some work around HIV/AIDS, don't think that you can just refer to preexposure prophylaxis as PrEP in your personal statement. The reader won't necessarily understand to what you are referring. You want to avoid slowing down the reader. As soon as they have to slow down to try to understand what you are trying to say, you'll start to lose them.

Don't bring in abbreviations from other parts of your application. If you defined MGH as Massachusetts General Hospital in your extracurriculars, don't just use MGH in your personal statement without defining it there as well. Don't force the reader to look up something he or she might not know.

Nontraditional Career Changers

If you're a nontraditional career changer, it is very common to write about why you are leaving your former career. As a reader, I'm not concerned about why you are leaving your old career; I want to know why you are excited to be starting a new one.

Again, *why do you want to be a physician,* not *this is why I don't want to be a computer programmer.*

It is very easy to bring negativity into a story about leaving your prior career, but you should avoid this at all costs. Writing about a bad boss, poor experiences, etc., will just show me that you are a complainer who will probably complain about things as a medical student and physician as well.

Look at this example from a student writing about why he's going into medicine:

I have chosen to pursue medicine due to a calling to assist people in a more meaningful and fulfilling way.

First of all, helping people in a meaningful and fulfilling way can be accomplished in thousands of different careers. Secondly, this is more of a complaint aimed at his current career. His current career isn't meaningful. His current career isn't fulfilling.

This is a very common phrase that students use—not being fulfilled. I'll caution you about referring to "not being fulfilled" because, at the end of the day, if you are looking for something external to fulfill you, you may be searching for that for the rest of your life.

Here is a good example of a student adding to his story about why he was a nontraditional, career-changing student:

Working full time throughout my undergraduate studies in order to support my wife and daughter slowed my educational progress and extended my timeline and path to my goal, but my desire to serve others never wavered.

I took a job at a healthcare information system company so that I could support my wife's educational goals and provide a stable income for our family while remaining close to medicine. It took seven long years to arrive at this point, but the time and circumstances now allowed me to commence on my journey.

He's not saying anything negative about his old career. He's just giving me a brief piece of information about it. It shows me that he is responsible, has a family, is probably organized, and can handle the stress of a lot of different responsibilities at the same time.

CHAPTER ELEVEN

WRITING FOR DIFFERENT APPLICATION SERVICES

Nothing about the premed journey is easy, and the application process is no different. There is an application service for osteopathic medical schools (AACOMAS), one for allopathic medical schools (AMCAS), and one for Texas (TMDSAS).

Some students apply to all three, some to only one. If you are planning to apply to all three, the question then becomes, do you have to write an essay for each application service? The answer is yes, and no.

Yes, because each application service has different character limits and if you write your first draft of your personal statement for the AMCAS application, which allows the most characters at 5,300, you're going to have to shorten it by 300 and 800 characters for the TMDSAS and AACOMAS applications, respectively.

No, because the goal for each of the application services is to describe your journey and what brought you to applying to medical school. That story isn't going to change between each of the application services.

The reason you want to be a physician, and what you hope to accomplish as a physician, are going to be the same no matter what medical school you go to.

Should I Write One Essay for the Shortest Character Count and Use that One Everywhere

Another very common question is a trick that some students use. They write an essay that is 4,500 characters in length, which is the maximum length for the AACOMAS essay. They then use this essay for the TMDSAS and AMCAS essays since the character count is below the other two.

This is possible, but may be viewed as lazy by some Admissions Committees looking at the TMDSAS and AMCAS essays. An essay that is 800 characters short stands out easily and the reason for why it is so short is obvious.

Use the extra characters allowed in the TMDSAS and AMCAS applications to your advantage. *Show* me one more experience that has strengthened your motivation to become a physician. Expand on your hopes for the future once you are a physician.

Don't cheat yourself out of your ability to separate yourself by not using as many characters as possible.

Do I Need to Write Specifically About Osteopathic Medicine?

This is one of the biggest questions that arises when writing a personal statement for the AACOMAS application. With osteopathic medical schools fighting every day to increase their awareness (yes, there are plenty of premeds who still don't know what a DO is), and their legitimacy (yes, there are plenty of (usually) older physicians who think that going to a DO school means you weren't smart enough to get into an MD school), some students feel like it is necessary to write specifically about why they want to go to an osteopathic medical school.

If you can do this naturally, meaning you've had some experience with DOs, and you can say that those moments have specifically caused you to pursue becoming an osteopathic medical student, then go ahead. Try to fit that extra story into the 800 fewer characters that you have from the AMCAS essay.

What you don't want to do is just randomly throw in the word *osteopathic* everywhere you refer to medical school and becoming a physician. This tactic just seems forced and inauthentic.

Here is an example of that:

I spoke with doctors, attended appointments, relayed sensitive information, provided wound care, and organized her treatment plans at home. This role was a natural fit—I found a sense of purpose in managing her care and a developing interest in osteopathic medicine as I gained more exposure to the medical field.

This student was discussing experiencing and interacting with the medical field after her mother suffered a massive heart attack. She states that she developed an interest in *osteopathic* medicine as she gained exposure to the medical field. This was very early on in her personal statement, and osteopathic medicine wasn't mentioned before. There was no mention of interacting with DOs. She didn't mention if an osteopathic physician treated her mom. Putting *osteopathic* into this sentence sounds forced. It continued throughout the rest of her personal statement. Read her final draft, SR Final Draft, in full in Section II of this book.

CHAPTER TWELVE

HOW TO EDIT YOUR PERSONAL STATEMENT

Getting feedback on your personal statement is the key to crafting your best story. Just like reviewing your full-length MCAT practice tests is the key to doing well on the MCAT, reviewing your personal statement at every step of the draft process is what will guarantee a better end product than just writing your essay and submitting it.

Many students don't know what to look for or who to ask for help when it comes to reviewing personal statements. That's what we'll cover here.

Editing for Story versus Editing for Grammar

One of the first things you should know is that your personal statement needs to be reviewed in two completely separate processes before you get to your final draft.

Editing your personal statement for its message is the most important edit that you can do. This isn't a one-time edit either. You need to perform an edit after every draft to make sure that the message you are actually delivering is what you intend to say. It's amazing how many times I write a comment on a personal statement and the students say, "That's not at all what I meant to say!" How you read what you wrote, and how someone else reads it, can be completely different.

Remember the goal of your message is to explain why you want to be a physician. If you hand your essay to a stranger, he or she should be able to tell you, in their own words, why you want to be a physician.

Editing for grammar should be the last step of the process. Once you are convinced that your personal statement has done its job of showing the reader why you want to be a physician, find someone who is a grammar expert. Get them to read through the essay and make sure that there are no typos, that the punctuation is correct, and that there are no other small mistakes.

Who to Turn to for Feedback

There are many people who you can turn to for feedback. Some have some drawbacks, and I'll discuss that here.

Premed Advisor

If you have access to your premed advisor, he or she is the first person you should get advice from on your personal statement. Your advisorresume should be the first person you go to for everything related to the premed path.

Depending on the volume of students the advising office sees at your school, there may be some hoops you have to jump through to get your personal statement reviewed, but usually, they are minimal and worthwhile.

If your advising office has restrictions on who they will see—i.e., students with above certain GPAs and MCAT scores—and you don't meet those minimums, you will need to seek guidance from friends, family, mentors, or private advisors.

Friends and Family

Turning to your friends and family is usually an easy option for most students. But do they *know* what they are looking at? Can they look at your personal statement objectively? Is your mom just going to be so proud of you that whatever you put in front of her is gold and will end up on the refrigerator?

It is important to get valuable, critical feedback. You're not looking to get praise at every step of the way. You want people to challenge you—to question what you are writing and why you are writing about it. Did you write an amazing first draft? Maybe. But it's not likely.

You want the person reading the essay to understand why you have chosen to pursue this path, and what you think your goals are for the future. You want them to feel some of the emotions that you felt along your journey. You don't want them to see just *what* you have done; you want them to know *why*.

To make sure that your friends and family are looking at your personal statement from the perspective of an advisor or even an Admissions Committee member, I created a review sheet that you can give them. You can download our 'Guide to Reviewing Personal Statements' at personalstatementbook.com/reviewsheet.

Physician Mentors

Physicians may be helpful in reviewing your personal statement. They have been through the process themselves and probably got feedback on their personal statements along the way.

Even though they have been through the process, though, this doesn't mean that they understand what Admissions Committees are looking for now. They may have an understanding of what worked for *them* but may not have the best feedback for your specific situation.

A physician will definitely be able to give you feedback on your core message regarding why you want to be a physician. They've been to medical school. They're practicing (or have practiced) as a physician, so they'll be able to see through any glaring issues with your *why*.

Remember that physicians are busy people. Be polite and give them a little extra time to review your personal statement. (The same applies if you're looking for a letter of recommendation. Usually the physicians take the longest.)

Review Swaps

If you go onto any premed forum online, you'll likely find a thread dedicated to review swaps. Students post and say that they have a personal statement for you to read, and in return, they will read yours.

My general rule of thumb is that review swaps should be your last resort. These students are very similar to your friends and family. You have to ask yourself, "Do they know *how* to give me feedback and *what* to give me feedback on? Do they know what a good *why* looks like?"

I do admit that I am a little more biased in this area because of the trend of cutthroat and negative attitudes on the same sites where students are performing swaps. The whole "premeds helping premeds with information they learned from other premeds" approach just doesn't make sense to me. It's the reason I started the Medical School Headquarters in 2012 and why I put out free podcasts every week. You can find them at mededmedia.com.

When preparing to write this book, I asked students to send me their essays and the feedback they received from student reviewers. Most of the feedback was grammatical in nature. There were a few good comments from one specific reviewer. The rest of the reviews were very generic and unhelpful.

If you are going to use a review swap, use the same review sheet that you can give your family and friends. You can download it at personalstatementbook.com/reviewsheet.

Professional Editing

There is no shortage of companies looking to help you edit your personal statement. It seems like every year, newly minted medical students start up a website and start offering their own service as well.

Don't get me wrong; I'm not saying they are bad. My company, Medical School Headquarters, also does personal statement editing.

Personal statement editing from a professional service can provide you with valuable feedback.

Here's what you should be looking for:

- A company that has inside knowledge about what medical schools are looking for. Just because someone is in medical school or is a resident doesn't mean they *know*.
- A company that has a track record of success, not just from students who have been accepted into medical school (since getting in is multifactorial), but can give you testimonials demonstrating that their students' personal statements have received great feedback from the Admissions Committees.
- A company that gives you at least two rounds of edits. You want to be able to make edits based on the feedback and get more feedback based on those edits to make sure you are headed in the right direction.
- A company that will let you ask questions based on the feedback they gave you. Sometimes there may be some misunderstanding or a clarification that needs to be made. Emailing with the reviewer, or jumping on a call, can quickly alleviate that.

Here's what you should completely avoid:
- A company that will write your personal statement for you. I've seen some students make "miraculous" strides with their personal statement, only to find out that it really wasn't their writing. This is against the rules for the application services and can get you in huge trouble if it's questioned at any point in the process. Unless you also pay for someone to write all of your secondary essays (which I'm not advocating for either), you are going to have a completely different style of writing and different voice between the primary and secondary applications.

Professional personal statement editing can be expensive for most students, so you should only consider it if it fits your budget.

If you have a great premed advisor whom you've learned to trust and with whom you have a great relationship, use him or her. If you have some great mentors in your life who are willing to give you some feedback, use them. If you don't have those, or if you still lack confidence in your personal statement, then looking into professional editing may be a good next step.

What to Do with Feedback After an Edit?

After every round of feedback, you need to figure out where you are going. Just like getting directions from a GPS, you need to figure out your route and from where you are starting.

With writing a personal statement, everyone is trying to end up in roughly the same location: showing the Admissions Committee why you want to be a physician. There will some small deviations based on your past. For instance, if you've had some major red flags, you will likely want to include that. A student who doesn't have red flags won't include those kinds of details. You'll probably also want to incorporate some statement regarding your future; what you hope to accomplish with the education that the medical school is going to give you.

Even though the ending is the same, the route will be completely different for each student. Each new draft gives you a new starting point, and each piece of feedback will hopefully redirect you to the proper route to tell *your* best story.

When you receive your feedback, reread your personal statement first, without looking at the reviewer's comments. This will bring the material back fresh to your mind. Ask yourself the same questions the reviewer was asking. Did this show the reader why I want to be a doctor? Did I write too much about extracurriculars or list my experiences like a résumé? Go down the list of questions so you can be prepared for the reviewer's comments.

If you're honest with yourself, you'll welcome each piece of feedback. You'll see every comment as a way to get your personal statement back on track to be the perfect personal statement that tells *your* story.

Sometimes you may disagree with the reviewer. That's okay. Maybe they misunderstood something, and you can clarify that. Maybe they are trying to tell you that you *need* to add something to your personal statement and you don't want to. First, make sure that what they are suggesting you add is actually your story, and not some generic statement. You'll need to ask them *why* they think it belongs—how will it add to your personal statement?

You may feel completely uncomfortable adding some of their suggestions into your personal statement, or, on the flip side, removing something from your personal statement. If you feel, at your core, that you have to have a certain piece of information in your personal statement, then put it in there. Just remember that what you are adding shouldn't be because you *think* it's what the Admissions Committee wants to read.

Drastic Changes Between Edits

Hopefully, after reading this book, your first draft is one that is on the right track to something great. It may be 10,000 characters and have poor grammar and punctuation, but it tells your story. If that is the case, then each subsequent draft is just about refining the message. You'll be cutting out characters, moving around stories, homing in on the closing, etc.

If you're way off base after your first draft, and you receive some good, constructive criticism, you may want to start fresh. If that's the case, go back and reread the chapters regarding what to write about and how to start your personal statement. Encouragement to start with a clean slate is a common piece of feedback that I give to students.

If you think you need to start again, don't worry. You're not alone. A large percentage of students who send me essays get the feedback to start over.

Final Edits

The final edits of your personal statement should be very nitpicky details that probably aren't going to affect your personal statement in large ways.

For some students I work with, I've done as many as twelve or thirteen edits. By the end, I am reading the personal statement in a very different way. The core message is already solid at that point, and I'm looking at things from a new angle. Take this sentence for example:

> *My imagination twisted the young woman into my mother, a nervous 36-year-old. Stomach churning, I relived the fear and sadness that permeated the kitchen when my mom told us she was dying.*

I left a comment that I was confused. Who was 36? The student's mom? Or the patient the student was writing about?

The final edit massaged it just a little bit to remove any confusion:

My mind brought me back to when my mom, in her late 30s, sat us down and told us she was dying from breast cancer.

In the draft, the student tried to get a little fancy with "imagination twisted" and "stomach churning." In the final draft, the reader can quickly understand what the student is saying without stopping to think about it.

Here is another small massage during the final edit stage.

The same student from the example above had this:

I lived for several weeks with a colleague, Steve, who spoke passionately about how their son's doctors changed their lives.

The message that followed was a great story about an experience that led to the student wanting to continue down her path. But something about "lived" stuck in my head as a potential issue for someone reading it. I asked her if it was really necessary to include that small detail? It wasn't. She changed it to this:

Around this time, my colleague often spoke passionately about how his son's doctors changed the lives of his family.

It says the same exact thing, and it does it without a potential red flag being raised.

In the next chapter, we'll talk about the final stage and how you know when you're truly done.

CHAPTER THIRTEEN

HOW TO KNOW IT'S FINALLY DONE

A premed and his or her personal statement are an inseparable couple until the very end. You could continue to tweak and edit your personal statement for years. You would never get anywhere though. At some point, good enough is all you need.

That doesn't mean that one draft is good enough. You still need to go through the editing process I described in the previous chapter.

If you can hand your personal statement to a stranger and ask them four questions, and they can give you the answers you were expecting, then you've done your job with your personal statement.

Here are the four questions that you should ask:

1) After reading my personal statement, can you tell me what my initial motivation was for exploring healthcare?

2) After reading the experiences I wrote about, can you tell me why they were important enough to put in my personal statement?

3) After reading my personal statement, do you see me doing anything else other than becoming a physician?

4) After reading my personal statement, what do you think I hope to accomplish as a physician?

If the answers you receive are what you expect, then you have probably written a great personal statement that will show the Admissions Committee why you want to be a doctor and what you hope to accomplish.

If you don't get the answers you expected, take the feedback and go back to the drawing board.

The personal statement writing process should be lengthy. Don't get frustrated if it's taking longer than *you* think it should take. I'd probably tell you that it's going to take three to four times longer than you expect.

As soon as you think it's good to go, put it aside. Don't look at it again. Don't even think about having someone else look at it. Once you have properly gone through the process of planning, writing, editing, and rechecking your work, you need to be done with it. Continuing to check your essay will just cause unneeded stress, anxiety, and fear.

Once you are done, start working on the secondary essay prompts. You want to get as much of a head start as possible.

At the end of the day, you have to remember that your personal statement is your story. Treat it with respect, just as you treat yourself with respect. You may need to write about potentially vulnerable experiences that expose aspects of your life that you don't usually like to talk about. That's okay.

If at the end of the process, including getting the good, constructive feedback you need, you feel like you've told your story, then you've done your job. Now focus on the rest of your application and click submit as soon as you can.

PERSONAL STATEMENT EXAMPLES FEEDBACK

A NOTE

I have obtained permission from every student for every personal statement example in this section. Some were personal statements that I personally edited and on which I gave direct feedback. Others were personal statements that were sent to me when I was looking for examples for this book. These personal statements are mostly unchanged, including any typos or grammatical errors, except for any personal details which were changed to keep students as anonymous as possible.

Not One Size Fits All

There are personal statements in here that were sent to me for this book, on which I gave some pretty thorough feedback. That doesn't mean they were bad personal statements; it just means that I would have liked to see something different to make them even stronger.

Who are They?

Unlike some other books with personal statements from all Ivy league students, the essays in this book are from students of all shapes and sizes going to both MD and DO schools throughout the country. These students didn't get an interview just because they had perfect grades and MCAT scores; they were invited because they had great stories. There are a couple personal statements from students still in the application cycle who haven't received acceptances yet.

My Feedback

After almost every paragraph, I have given you my direct feedback regarding the preceding text. Because it's been some time since I've given feedback on some of these personal statements, my advice to the student and my feedback now may be a little different. That's the frustrating thing about writing personal statements—the reader's perspective and thoughts are constantly changing based on their interactions with the world and other personal statements they have read. You can't control that, so you just need to focus on writing *your* best personal statement.

MY PERSONAL STATEMENT

The doctor and assistant suited up, strapping what looked like fanny packs onto their waists to sanitize the air they breathed. Blue suits wrapped their bodies, connecting to matching helmets, while latex gloves hugged their hands. I watched, as they stepped through the doors into a world into which I had never ventured. Since I was not going to be near the patient, I did not need to wear a suit. I knocked on the doors to operating room number nine where a total knee replacement was ready to be implanted, awaiting approval for my entrance.

Once I got in room nine, I watched as the doctor approached the steel table draped with blue sheets and began discussing his next steps. He called for more drapes, for the tourniquet to be inflated, and for a knife to start the two-hour long procedure. The confidence and calmness of a person that has another one's life in their hands was remarkable. This was the first of many experiences observing surgery, and seeing how one human being can directly affect another's life was what strengthened my resolve to pursue a career as a physician.

My first upclose exposure to the world of medicine came with the death of my father. A Friday-night phone call while I was sleeping informed me that he was in the hospital after a brain aneurysm; that phone call changed the path of my life. I stayed by his bedside for two days, watching in awe as the doctors and nurses came and went, not showing any outwardly signs of the pressure they faced every day. As busy as they were and as quickly as they worked, they always had time to take care of my father and answer my family's questions. I wondered what role I could play in other people's lives so they would not have to go through what I was experiencing.

An elective class during my senior year of high school followed, Anatomy and Physiology, leading to my overwhelming interest in the intricacies of the human body. I learned about all systems of the body from the text, before using cow and sheep parts to study them up close. The rest of the class was devoted to the dissection of a cat; I was nicknamed "the cat man" for my relentless pursuit of perfection in the dissection of "Mr. Bigglesworth." The dissection experience sharpened my interest in medicine, and I realized that not just medicine, but surgery, was in my future. A trip to Kenya, East Africa, after high school, opened my eyes to helping people outside medicine.

I worked at an orphanage called "Nyumbani" (Swahili for "home"), the only orphanage in Kenya with hospice services and healthcare for HIV + infants and children. My weekdays were spent doing manual labor in the main reception and hospital sections, but my most rewarding time was spent playing with the kids. If I had a free hand when I was walking through the playground, it was only because none of the children had reached me yet. It was here that I learned that the combination of medical school and humanitarian experience would make me the best doctor that I could be.

With these goals in mind, I began following a physician in August, 2002 after my move to Colorado. Observing the rigorous daily schedule of a surgeon has given me new insight into the realities and rigors of surgery, not scaring me away but convincing me that I am in the right place. From eight to five, I stand side by side with the doctor as he tells patients the good news and bad. Never has a patient refused to let me observe an exam; they know, as I do, that the future of medicine relies on students like me.

Each visit I make to the doctor's office confirms my career choice, teaching me more and more, and I go home each day looking forward to the next. When I received the letters from my first attempts at application medical school, I was reminded of my shoulder injury in high school. The many trips to the physical therapist taught me that goals in this life are met only through sheer determination and perseverance. The American poet Henry Wadsworth Longfellow wrote, "Perseverance is a great element of success. If you only knock long enough and loud enough at the gate, you are sure to wake up somebody." I have begun my knocking, and I look forward to walking through the door just as I did on that day several months ago when I entered the operating room number nine and seeing all there is to see in medicine.

AK EARLY DRAFT

My eight years as an Army officer were the defining experience of my life. I joined ROTC shortly after 9/11, proud to serve the people of the country I loved. The recruiter told me that as an officer I would be in a unique position of influence and responsibility, granted an opportunity to do just what the commercials said: to "be all that you can be."

> *Here, the student is telling me about 9/11 and joining the ROTC. It was very bland and didn't engage me.*

Years later in Afghanistan, I had the opportunity to do just that. My mission was to lead our unit's tactical operations center, planning and tracking all movements of our personnel and orchestrating the unit's response in the case of unexpected events. Mistakes had real-world consequences, and with a small margin for error, every day required a firstrate effort. It was the first time in my life I had felt in flow—receiving reports, making decisions, and issuing orders. I loved it.

> *Again, the student is just explaining what is happening.*

The urgency of our mission hit home during Operation Proper Exit, a program to return horrifically injured soldiers, now physically healed, to the site of their trauma in an effort to heal the invisible wounds of PTSD. I had the opportunity to meet these soldiers who, despite debilitating burns and lost limbs, were incredibly grateful to be alive. The timely work of trauma teams and enduring efforts of medical care providers had taken away the pain and had given them their lives back.

> *Here, we're finally starting to get some medical aspects creeping in, which is good.*

Sharing in their experience compelled me to reflect on my life as an officer. While I impacted lives, it paled in comparison to the tireless medical labors that had saved these soldiers. This was the type of significance I wanted my life to have: to nurture the living, heal for the sick, and comfort the distressed. It spoke to the core of my being.

> *The paragraph starts with the takeaway from the previous paragraph. The takeaway is important—why are you telling me this?*

I would stay in the military an additional three years to accomplish my ultimate goal upon joining the Army: being a company commander. Command was the most humbling experience of my life. Both my superiors and subordinates, Japanese and American, trusted me to execute complex missions and issue orders that were legally, morally, and ethically sound. Deciding how to rule on inherently gray situations, unraveling the tug-of-war between several sides of a story, that would impact and, in some cases, end careers was the greatest challenge I have confronted. As I completed my command and military commitment, the time had arrived to pursue my dream of a career in medicine.

> *This paragraph is just a snippet of a biography, a piece of the student's résumé that doesn't need to be in the personal statement. The student is trying to highlight that he executed "complex missions" and issued "orders that were legally, morally, and ethically sound." Remember, you don't need to sell your skills and traits. This isn't the purpose of the personal statement.*

Upon being honorably discharged, I moved back to my hometown to attend State University. Far from the boy that arrived at college twelve years prior, I returned to academia as a grown man with renewed focus and maturity. The intervening years on the battlefield had equipped me with the tenacity and determination to pursue my aspiration of becoming a doctor. At State University, my lifelong interest in how the world worked became a fascination with science as I sought and devoured knowledge both in and out of the classroom. Applying these principles while researching the biological impacts of medically promising nanoparticles both furthered my transition from soldier to scientist and familiarized me with the organization and skillful coordination required for multi-institutional projects.

> *This continues the resume or timeline writing that should be removed from your writing. You don't need to chronicle each step of the way.*

Beyond the classroom, volunteering in my local emergency department played a central role in validating my passion for medicine. Rounding on patients, classroom lessons were given real-world context as I learned about the health issues confronting my community. Discussing ailments with patients only to learn they were not taking their medications despite being desperate to regain their health did not initially make sense. But then learning about the physical and psychological side effects related to the treatment brought the complexity and challenges of effective health management to life. When patients confronted these frightening scenarios and the grayness of what was actually happening, it was their doctor they turned to for guidance.

> *This is another paragraph of the student* telling *me about an experience. It could have been much stronger if he had painted the picture of an interaction with a patient who was turning to their doctor for guidance.*

Time and again, I have found that my most meaningful clinical experiences stem not from observing a prescription of treatment, but instead arise from this implicit partnership between patient and physician. This relationship is unique in that patients regularly entrust people they have just met with their health and often their lives. At their most vulnerable moments, patients fully commit themselves to the skill, knowledge, and compassion of their physician. It is this special relationship that distinguishes doctors among healthcare providers, the innate trust of a patient to follow doctor's orders.

> *This is an example of the student telling me what being a doctor is like. Just because you know what being a doctor is like, doesn't mean you should become one.*

This trust reminds me of my most valued interactions as an officer. Soldiers trust that their leaders are inherently working in their best interests with a high level of expertise, competence, and professionalism. Fulfilling this unwritten contract is what fueled me through long days in Afghanistan and compelled me to pursue my graduate, linguistic, and technical education on nights and weekends while in uniform. This drive—to develop myself to better serve my patients—will give me the determination to overcome the challenges presented by medical school and residency. Each morning I wake up resolved to become a reliable, competent doctor worthy of that supreme trust and capable of changing lives like those of the soldiers we welcomed back to Afghanistan six years ago.

> *Remember what I said at the beginning about the student trying to sell me his skills? He wasn't explicitly making the connections before, but now he's really trying to drive them home.*
> *After reading this, I told the student that he needed to rewrite it, focusing on increasing the amount of showing and not telling. I think he started with the right ideas and had good experiences; he just needed to reframe them. You can read the final draft next.*

AK FINAL DRAFT

As the sun set in Afghanistan and the buzz of floodlight generators filled the air, my commander and I arrived at the Armored Division headquarters. Amid the sea of digital camouflage, high and tight haircuts, and matte black steel, the honorees of the evening awaited. Having been horrifically wounded and now physically healed, they were returning to the site of their traumas in an effort to heal the invisible wounds of PTSD. It was hard not to stare given their injuries—missing limbs, burn scars, or in some cases nothing apparent aside from a look in their eyes. But within our gazes was a common understanding that this could have happened to any of us, and for many, had happened to people we knew. The soldiers told their stories to the quieted audience, stories that began similarly to any of our days. Within each of their tales was an overwhelming gratefulness for the timely work of trauma teams and the enduring medical efforts during rehabilitation. Their names were not mentioned but the importance of their work apparent to all, and for me set in motion the pursuit of a career in medicine.

As you start this personal statement, you're immediately hit with some visuals that get your senses going. "Missing limbs, burn scars" and the "look in their eyes" are all great showing phrases. The student paints the picture so that I feel like I'm there with him.

These doctors had saved lives, taken away the pain, and given their patients hope despite their hardships. Walking back into the desert night to my bunk, I could not stop thinking about what I had just encountered. Sharing in this experience compelled me to reflect on my life as an officer. Shortly after 9/11, I joined the Army to ensure the vulnerability and pain I felt that day would never be repeated. By training our team for deployment and organizing missions in Afghanistan, I felt I was fulfilling this promise. While I impacted the lives of my soldiers and contributed to the wartime mission, the outcomes paled in comparison to the tireless medical labors that had saved the soldiers I had just met. This was the type of significance I wanted my life to have: to nurture the living, to heal for the sick, and to comfort the distressed. Never before had I felt this draw to medicine, but the human impact of talking to soldiers who in many ways should not have been alive spoke to the core of my being.

This draw persisted throughout the deployment and into my next assignment, the seminal position of company command. The experience would take me to Japan for over two years that indelibly influenced my understanding of leadership and professionalism. As the assignment neared completion and I approached the possibility of a lifelong military career, I examined my values, experiences, and goals, and my decision to pursue medicine was clear and wholehearted.

> *These two paragraphs are a little long for a career change statement, but it works well. It tells me why the student is switching careers. It shows great personal reflection.*

After being honorably discharged, I returned to my hometown to attend State University. Whereas my previous undergraduate experience had been a chore on the way to my mission, school was now the compelling force in my life. With studies focused on the function of the body, hours of study passed without notice as my appetite for knowledge continually increased. Volunteering at my local emergency department (ED) gave me the opportunity to interact with patients and care providers and witness the human side of medicine.

> *This paragraph doesn't tell me much and probably could have been cut to make room for another story.*

Upon arrival at the ED, patients entrusted their well-being to a team of care providers they had never met before in a wholly unfamiliar environment replete with beeping monitors, scents of surface disinfectants, and people in variously colored scrubs moving about in every direction. My role within the ED was to familiarize the patients with their surroundings, ask about their care, and comfort them when needed. Characteristic of my experience was encountering a patient alone and deeply distraught over two broken fingers, a response that seemed out of place until finding they were a professional violinist. While a splint would eventually set their fingers, telling them that bones heal and everything would be okay visibly contributed to their overall condition. The satisfaction I derived from these small contributions made it clear I was pursuing a heartfelt goal. Commonly, I discovered patients lacked knowledge on how lifestyle affected health, basic facts that may have improved their lives. These lessons motivated me to join Americorps for my upcoming glide year, selected to be a health and life skills educator for the homeless of northern Florida.

> *The description of being with someone who broke their fingers and finding out they were a professional violinist was great. I could picture the student being there, listening, and showing empathy. He didn't have to* tell *me he was empathetic; he did it with his writing. There is also a great takeaway with his statement about how it was "clear I was pursuing a heartfelt goal." The last statement probably could have been cut since it's just a generic extracurricular statement.*

From these candid patient interactions I also came to understand their basic expectations of honesty, respect, and expert care from their physicians while in their most vulnerable moments. Stripped down to a hospital gown and in pain, often without a known cause, it was inevitably their doctor to whom our patients looked for guidance when making life-altering decisions. This trust reminds me of soldiers trusting that their leaders are inherently working in their best interests with a high level of expertise, competence, and professionalism. Fulfilling this unwritten contract is what fueled me through long days in Afghanistan. This drive—to develop myself to better serve my patients—will give me the determination to overcome the challenges presented by medical school and residency. Each morning I wake up resolved to become a reliable, competent doctor worthy of that supreme trust, capable of changing lives like those of the soldiers we welcomed back to Afghanistan six years ago and the patients who visit doctors every day.

This conclusion retains some of the qualities that the student wanted to leave in about being a military officer. One thing to keep in mind, going back to the draft, is even though I recommended removing some of the selling type statements, the student thought this was important enough to include. Ultimately, I think he had a good argument to leave it in. As a former military officer, he's going to be a unique candidate and wanted me to have a little insight into what skills he gained from that experience. At the end of the day, you have to be comfortable with what is in your personal statement or what you take out of your personal statement.

This final draft came from a couple of rounds of edits. Compare this to his early draft on the previous page. See if you can spot the differences between showing *and* telling. *This student was accepted to several allopathic medical schools and is now attending an Ivy league medical school.*

AC FIRST DRAFT

As a new volunteer at the free clinic, I sat in the corner of the exam room and observed an experienced volunteer begin an intake for a new patient. The patient was a young man with a couple of cracked front teeth, sitting opposite me with his uncle. I silently listened to the other volunteer ask the patient for basic contact information while thinking that this guy couldn't even bother to take care of teeth let alone his overall health. I was soon proven very wrong as the story of his life and health unfolded. The young man was only nineteen years old; he had cracked his teeth in a fast food restaurant, his face hitting the counter when he lost consciousness during an epileptic seizure. The boy's parents were drug addicts and often not present, the only person in his life he could rely on was his uncle. At this point during the intake the other volunteer stopped what he was doing, got up, walked over to the uncle, shook his hand and said, "Thank you." I learned two very important lessons that day. First, that there is no place for judgment and jumping to conclusions in healthcare; and second, the importance of a support system and the significance of acknowledging its importance.

> *The student opens up by describing one of her shadowing experiences. I was excited to see this in a first draft! But after reading the takeaway—don't judge or jump to conclusions and the value of a support system—I was confused as to why she was telling me these things. The question I often respond to students with is, "Why does this make you want to be a physician?" Not being judgmental and jumping to conclusions is great for every career. Heck, it's a great trait for every human.*

I volunteered at this clinic for a year where I gained practical clinical skills, such as taking vitals and writing a progress note, but it also provided exposure to a diverse group of patients. Be that these people did not have health insurance; they came from all walks of life. The patients ranged from graduate students to drug addicts, illegal immigrants to recently unemployed. One patient, an older gentleman, was frequenting the clinic due to his uncontrolled diabetes. The physician he saw at the clinic was present one day a week the same day that I was and so I often interacted with this patient. Every other week or so, I would see this man, I grew accustomed to pricking his coarse hands at the fingertip for the glucometer, which one day maxed out and could not give me a number. Therefore, I questioned the man about what he had to eat and drink that day. He obliged, he hadn't eaten much in the past few hours but he drank a Gatorade on his way to clinic which he proceeded to tell me was ok because it wasn't sweet. I finally realized the root of his inability to control his blood sugars, a lack of education on the disease and nutrition. After this, I sat down with him and some sample nutrition labels and went over the importance of and how to read the labels.

> *This is another good example of a story with no takeaway. Why are you telling me this? Why is this important? Don't force me to figure it out. Let me know why this experience was so important that you decided to include it in your personal statement and how it confirmed your decision to become a physician.*

I cannot pinpoint a particular moment in time or experience that first influenced my decision to become a physician, but rather my journey has snowballed as I have gained education and experience of the practice. High school biology provided the first of many astonishing discoveries; I can recall the day I learned about cancer. Prior to this, I possessed a vague concept of it as a big scary disease, but when I learned that it originated from our very own cells, I was floored. That evening I told my mother what I had found out that day and to my dismay she was not surprised.

Putting the origin story about why medicine *so deep in the personal statement is burying the most important part of your story. This* IS *her origin story. This is the spark, or the "seed," as I've talked about previously. This needs to be the start of her personal statement. This is what started the snowball.*

A career in medicine is a commitment to lifelong learning. This continual intellectual stimulation is a factor that has drawn me into this career, but even more so, the prospect of contributing to it. As an undergraduate student I worked in a molecular genetics research laboratory and currently I work as a clinical research coordinator specifically for cystic fibrosis studies. My passion within medicine lies in research. I want to contribute to the understanding of the human body and I want to make an impactful improvement in people's lives. The breadth of possibility within research creates an environment to more readily make that impact. It is an exciting time to be in medicine where so many resources are at our fingertips yet, as said by a previous professor of mine, there is still so much we don't know and so much we don't know that we don't know.

This paragraph tells me that the student has done research and likes it. It's telling *me. If she included something about what she did, how it impacted her, or how she hopes to use it in the future, it would be better. I don't recommend comparing medicine to lifelong learning. To be good at anything in life means to be a lifelong learner.*

My premedical path has not been a traditional one, but it has certainly taught me a lot about myself and my chosen career path. I rounded out the first year of college with less than stellar grades. I recognize this was in part due to the novelty of being away from home and never really learning how to study. At this point, medical school was a distant goal for which I had not yet gained a real drive or passion. I was not even aware I could volunteer in a hospital until my sophomore year. It took some time beyond my undergraduate career to provide adequate academic and experiential evidence that I have chosen the right career path, but I am proud of the path I have taken. Without having taken this path I would not have had the pleasure of working in clinical research with individuals with cystic fibrosis. They are an inspiring patient population. The amount of time and effort they must put into their health every day in addition to leading normal, hectic everyday lives is remarkable, and then they still find the time to participate in clinical research. I am honored they allow me to poke and prod every detail of their health, often at no immediate benefit to them, in an attempt to move one step closer to finding a cure. As much as I love this work, I feel that I will not be fulfilled facilitating other people's ideas.

One quick note is the length of these paragraphs. They are very long. A typical English class will tell you that a paragraph should be four-five sentences. In today's Internet world, shorter paragraphs are ok.

In this paragraph, the student writes, "at this point." At what point? Before the bad grades or after? I could think about it for a second and figure out what she is telling me, but you don't want to force me to think like that. It slows me down.

She mentions taking some time for "experiential evidence" that she is supposed to be a physician. This is the exact goal of the personal statement. What were those experiences?

That's what I want to know about.

Check out her final draft next.

AC FINAL DRAFT

As a new volunteer at the free clinic, I sat in the corner of the exam room and observed an experienced volunteer begin an intake for a new patient. The patient was a young man with a couple of cracked front teeth, sitting opposite me with his uncle. I silently listened to the other volunteer ask for basic contact information while thinking that this guy couldn't even bother to take care of teeth let alone his overall health. I was soon proven very wrong as the story of his life and health unfolded. The young man was only nineteen years old; he had cracked his teeth in a fast food restaurant, his face hitting the counter when he lost consciousness during an epileptic seizure. The boy's parents were drug addicts and often not present, the only person in his life he could rely on was his uncle. At this point during the intake the other volunteer stopped what he was doing, got up, walked over to the uncle, shook his hand and said, "Thank you." Although I played no part in this encounter other than to observe, I soaked up so much more information beyond how to take a medical history. It was the first time I confronted the impact social factors could have on a person's health; and at that free clinic, it wouldn't be last.

> *The student opens up the personal statement in a very similar way to before, but she has changed her takeaway. It explains not judging and jumping to conclusions much better, but it's still not as strong as I would have liked. If I were reading this, I would ask: "Why not be a social worker then?" The takeaway isn't tied to medicine, so it's not as strong as it could be, but much improved over the first draft.*

My premedical path has not been a traditional one, but it has certainly taught me a lot about myself and my chosen career path. I rounded out the first year of college with less than stellar grades. I recognize this was in part due to the novelty of being away from home, never previously learning how to study, and not yet having a passion for medicine instilled in me. In an effort to redeem myself, I improved my grades, became involved in research, shadowed physicians, engaged in clinical volunteer work, continued academic pursuit, and found employment in healthcare settings. The prolonged premedical path I have taken has allowed me to ensure I have chosen the right career path and persevering through mistakes and setbacks has motivated me to obtain this goal.

> *This is a red flag paragraph. The student is trying to make me aware of why she has poor grades and what she did to improve them. It's a little long, at over 16% of the total character count, but it does what it needs to do.*

The continual intellectual stimulation and the necessity of staying up-to-date on information and advancements is a factor that has drawn me into this career, but even more so, the prospect of contributing to it. As a freshman in college I had no idea undergraduate students could conduct research. I thought that was something that was left to the professionals. But after going to a talk about research given by the biology department chairman, I decided I wanted to work in his lab. So I earned my way into his molecular genetics research laboratory and loved it. I spent all of my free time there. I, a lowly undergraduate student, was actually contributing to the knowledge of the human genome.

> *Writing about research can be a tricky proposition. Yes, research is an important aspect of the job, but it's just a small part for most physicians. The majority of physicians don't do research; they do clinical work and read others' research. Reading this paragraph makes me think: "Why not become a Ph.D. researcher?"*

When I worked as a hospital pharmacy technician, I had little to no patient contact and it was easy to fall into the service of the job: providing inventory to nurses. But when I would put on the protective gown and extra thick gloves to compound chemotherapy at the special hood for a patient my sister's age, I was reminded of the reality and gravity of the task at hand. This woman my sister's age was fighting a battle so great that I have to protect myself from the very therapy that treats her. I would remind myself that, if this were my sister I would want everyone carrying out their jobs as precisely as possible and I would carry this thought with me to every medication I prepared.

> *Bringing it back to patient care is great. Being around a patient and how it made the student feel is what I like to see. The takeaway could be stronger, tying it into her future as a physician and not just preparing medications. Again, I could ask: "Why not be a nurse, or pharmacist, or even stay a pharmacy technician?"*

Currently I work as a clinical research coordinator for Cystic Fibrosis studies. Most of my studies are clinical trials, which have exposed me to the process of translating knowledge gained from bench research into a clinical application. But what has truly astounded me is the community of clinicians and researchers dedicated to finding a cure. Conducting research in the Cystic Fibrosis community is not just a job or even a career; it's a way of life. The only thing I find more impressive than this community are the patients themselves. I am honored that they allow me to poke and prod every detail of their health with the goal of finding therapies that can benefit every individual with Cystic Fibrosis. I get to facilitate patients providing hope for themselves and others that one day we will find a cure.

> *The student describes another good story of patient exposure in this paragraph, but again, the takeaway isn't as strong as it could be. "I get to facilitate patients providing hope for themselves and others that one day we will find a cure." I still wonder: "Why not become a research coordinator?"*

Although I enjoy working as a clinical research coordinator, I would not be fulfilled pursuing this as a career. I need to be able contribute to our medical knowledge base through my own inquisition, not just by facilitating the ideas of others. I want to care for patients, not just study subjects; taking into consideration social factors that could affect their health like the boy at the free clinic and treat them as if I were taking care of my own family as the oncology patient had reminded me of my sister.

In this last paragraph, I am finally given some more information about why medicine, or better yet, why physician?
These pieces of information could have been much more effective if they were sprinkled throughout the essay and not just as the final paragraph. One question left is about her sister. The student mentioned her sister a couple of times but doesn't explain why she is writing about her.
I'm left to assume her sister had cancer, but don't know for sure.
Overall, this essay tells me what I need to hear, why medicine, but it could have been much more powerful with some tweaks.
This student is attending an osteopathic medical school in the Midwest.

AS FIRST DRAFT

Hepatic encephalopathy, pulmonary edema, hepatorenal syndrome, hospice. The doctor's words felt like a punch to my gut. Although my veterinary education allowed me to comprehend what was being said, my heart was not yet ready to accept the true meaning. I spent the days that followed at my father's bedside. His hospital room showed its age; white walls, chipped floor tiles, and a wall mounted heating unit intermittently groaning. The saving grace of the room was the single, large window that faced a greenbelt. My father had slipped into a coma before I arrived at the hospital, but I spoke to him anyway. I sang him songs that I thought might comfort him, and prayed he could hear me. I served as a makeshift interpreter for my extended family during the daily visits with his doctors. Some of the family remained hopeful that he would miraculously recover, but the doctors steadfastly repeated their list of diagnoses and the grave prognosis. In the end, the doctors had only been wrong about the transfer to a hospice facility. I held his hand as he drew his final breath on that cold December morning, still in the same hospital room, overlooking the beautiful evergreens. As I left the hospital that day, I felt for the first time a desire to become a physician.

This is a powerful opening that paints the picture of this student's father's death. It does a great job of showing me what was going on and the impact it had on her decision to be a physician. It's a great opening with a great takeaway.

As a newly minted veterinarian, I wrestled with the idea of changing paths. The road to becoming a veterinarian had not been easy. At the ripe old age of 21, I was a newlywed as well as a new mother. My husband and I struggled to support our small family and, for a time, even received support from the Women, Infants and Children nutrition program. At the time, my father was homeless due to a combination of alcoholism and mental illness, and we stretched even farther to support him as well. I often worked two or more jobs while attending college, which, not surprisingly, hurt my undergraduate grade point average. There were several times when I had to withdraw from classes in favor of work until we could afford for me to return once again. Through hard work and determination, I was eventually accepted to veterinary school.

> *This is a good red flag statement that also lets me know that the student is coming from another profession. It* shows *me how she struggled financially, even being on food stamps, and it tips me off that she is going to have some poor grades.*

Juggling the responsibilities of my family and the rigors of veterinary school tested my ability to efficiently manage my time as well as my resolve to reach that goal. Despite these challenges, I excelled in my training and graduated with honors. In the months after my father's death, I questioned whether it was even reasonable to ask my family to support me through medical school and the residency that would follow. Ultimately, the commitment I had already made to the United States Army Veterinary Corps forced me to set aside my aspirations of becoming a physician.

> *This is where the personal statement starts to lose me. This paragraph tells* me nothing about medicine, only that she served in the military as a veterinarian. This could easily be removed.*

The last seven years I have spent as a veterinarian have been very rewarding. Although many choose veterinary medicine to avoid working with people, I felt exactly the opposite. Certainly, I enjoy interacting with my animal patients, but I have always felt the greatest satisfaction from the opportunity to form a relationship with my patient's family. One particularly memorable patient was a kitten rushed in as an emergency one Saturday afternoon. The family had adopted the kitten from the local shelter just a day prior. On presentation, we observed that the kitten was in shock and lying in his kennel on top of a pile of his small intestines. Our team worked quickly to stabilize and prepare him for surgery. His injuries required me to perform a resection and anastomosis due to considerable damage to a portion of his intestine. Despite the severity of his injuries, he recovered beautifully from surgery and his family was overjoyed. The next time I saw the family their five-year-old daughter told me how much the kitten meant to her and thanked me for saving him. Naturally, I felt immense satisfaction for the role I played in the positive outcome for that patient and his family. However, those feelings were tempered by the lingering thoughts of how much more meaningful that same experience would be if my patient had instead been someone's mother, brother, or child. While my love of medicine has not changed, I find myself called to serve the people around me in a more direct way.

You can probably see that the student is trying to tie why medicine *into this paragraph by writing about saving a kitten, but wanting more and wanting it to be a human patient. From my perspective, it's just not a strong enough connection. She's talking about a kitten and not a human. They are two completely different things. At this point, I need to see how she has been around human patients.*

I am a person of faith and I believe that things happen for a reason. Had I initially sought acceptance to medical school rather than veterinary school, I would have missed many experiences that have been transformative in my life. The last decade has equipped me with greater perspective, emotional maturity and a stronger sense of purpose. I have learned how to counsel families regarding medical conditions and partner with them to find treatment plans that are best for their situation. Through my journey as a mother, I have found that I am particularly passionate about issues surrounding women's healthcare. I have learned to balance the demands of a service-focused career and the needs of my family. We are now financially and emotionally prepared for me to begin medical school. Most of all, I know that I have much more to learn in the years ahead. Although I am anything but a traditional applicant, I am confident that I can bring unique value to my medical school class and, someday, to my community as a physician.

The ending is nice, but when I am finished reading this, all I know is that the student really liked being a vet, but now she wants to be a physician. I don't know much more than that, other than the initial story of her father. As a reader, I'm left wondering if she will really enjoy being around human patients, or if she'll miss her furry friends instead. See her final draft on the next page.

AS FINAL DRAFT

Hepatic encephalopathy, pulmonary edema, hepatorenal syndrome, hospice. The doctor's words felt like a punch to my gut. Although my veterinary education allowed me to comprehend what was being said, my heart was not yet ready to accept the true meaning. I spent the days that followed at my father's bedside. His hospital room showed its age; white walls, chipped floor tiles, and a wall mounted heating unit intermittently groaning. The saving grace of the room was the single, large window that faced a greenbelt. My father had slipped into a coma before I arrived at the hospital, but I spoke to him anyway. I sang him songs that I thought might comfort him, and prayed he could hear me. I served as a makeshift interpreter of medical terminology for my extended family during the daily visits with his doctors. Some of the family remained hopeful that he would miraculously recover, but the doctors steadfastly repeated their list of diagnoses and the grave prognosis. In the end, the doctors had only been wrong about the transfer to a hospice facility. I held his hand as he drew his final breath on that cold December morning, still in the same hospital room, overlooking the beautiful evergreens. As I left the hospital that day, I felt the desire to become a physician begin to take root.

You can see that the opening didn't change much. It didn't need to. It's a strong opening that gives me the "seed" that was planted.

Over the years that followed my father's death, I tried to focus on my veterinary career. In the Army Veterinary Corps, I belonged to the Public Health Command. With that experience came a fair amount of exposure to human healthcare. I worked with physicians to help determine the human risk following potential rabies exposure situations. I received training in basic first aid as well as CPR certification. In addition, I attended a specialty course to help manage human casualties in the event of a nuclear, biological, or chemical disaster situation. While I was proud of my contribution in service to our country, I longed to be able to provide medical care to soldiers, rather than their pets. Despite this, I told myself that medical school was no longer an option for me; that the opportunity had somehow been extinguished with the candles on my thirtieth birthday cake. And yet, with each passing year my interest in becoming a physician has only grown. In 2016, my tipping point arrived in the form of a handsome baby boy named John.

Here, the student gives me some background info about her role in the Army and as a veterinarian. She was able to, unlike her previous draft, write about contact with human patients and working with physicians. She then gives a good transition to John. You don't need to worry about transitions too much. This isn't a formal writing project that needs smooth transitions at every point.

At 32 weeks into her pregnancy, a friend and fellow veterinarian received the devastating news that her son had Trisomy 18. She shared their family's journey through the many struggles, as well as the unexpected triumphs, of John's 135 days of life. He was hospitalized multiple times in his short life for congestive heart failure, infectious respiratory disease and pulmonary hypertension. Her stories left me feeling utterly helpless. Once again I found myself with enough knowledge to understand the extreme difficulty he faced but without any tangible way to impact his care. John was treated by a group of dedicated, caring physicians who helped his family navigate a path that no parent wants to walk. Without their expert care, John may not have even survived his birth. There is unspeakable beauty in that truth; that the work of his doctors gave his mother and father precious time to know their child. In witnessing this, I knew I could no longer set aside my dream of becoming a physician. I want to be able to be the person offering hope to patients in the face of illness and fear. I have come to realize that my prior experiences, both professional and as a wife and mother, are not a hindrance as I once thought, but rather a resource toward becoming an empathetic and relatable physician.

> *Here is a story of a human patient, a friend of the student, who needed care and left the student feeling helpless. Her takeaway is about empowering herself to make the transition to becoming a physician to care for human patients.*

At its best, I see medicine as a union of the science of healing with the mindful respect of the individual patient's needs. I have been fortunate to shadow a doctor that seems to do this with ease. One memorable patient was a middle-aged man frustrated by poor control of his type 2 diabetes. Upon further investigation, the doctor learned the patient was a truck driver. This made healthy eating habits and regular exercise challenging. Additionally, he was not taking his metformin because it caused diarrhea. By seeking to know his patient as an individual, the doctor was able to partner with the patient to develop alternate strategies to effectively manage his disease. This interaction is a perfect example of how I hope to practice medicine; an approach that is patient-centered and collaborative.

The student ends with one final story to wrap things up. She gives a brief "what do I want to do with my life" type finish. I think it could have given me a little bit more—a bigger idea, but it is okay. This submitted draft, versus the first draft, does a much better job of telling me more about why medicine. It tells me about the experiences that pushed her to continue on this journey. The first draft is mostly about being a veterinarian. This final draft is much more about why medicine.

AR EARLY DRAFT

I often hear, "You're crazy!" when my undergraduate peers learn that I have five kids, or when I tell a fellow mom that I'm applying to medical school. I realize I am a little out of the ordinary, but taking a nontraditional route to get where I want to be isn't crazy. In fact, it's second nature for me. After all, my life has been anything but traditional.

> *This is an interesting opening that tells me immediately that this student is nontraditional. It doesn't have to start with* **why medicine** *or a fancy story. It just needs to make me want to keep reading, which this one does.*

My interest in medicine began with my mother's illnesses. I was eight years old when she told me she had six months to live. I lived in fear of her death as she grew pale and thin. One day, my father was out of town as was common, she emerged from the bathroom, bald. She miraculously recovered, only to become gravely ill once again. Over the years, she studied from her Merck Manual and other texts about her conditions. She would explain her diseases to me: leukemia and brain tumors, a hole in her heart and fibromyalgia. I read over her shoulder and poured over the pages myself. I was fascinated by the human body and its parts and how they worked together. I was obsessed by how it could also go so very wrong, and why. In my high school biology class, I learned about genetics and the Human Genome project and I was enchanted that so much information could be packed into each cell. I never tired of biology and the more I learned, the more I wanted to know.

This is the seed. This paragraph sets the tone for the why. She shows me by saying, "I read over her shoulder and poured over the pages myself." If you remember earlier in this book when I mentioned counting the "I [verb]" statements, you might think that this paragraph is too telling. I would agree. It could be stronger with more showing, but it's still a good paragraph overall.

While this was the reality I experienced as a young person and this environment nourished my interest in the human body and science, many years later, I learned that my mother never had any of those diseases. They were a mask for her real disease, prescription drug addiction, which would eventually take her life.

When I first read this paragraph, I was amazed that everything that had just been told to me was not true. This plot twist is like something out of a good movie. I didn't see it coming, and it just piqued my interest even more.

I was 17 when I made my first nontraditional journey into postsecondary education. My friends were ending their junior year in high school, but I was impossibly behind. I had been kept home from high school to care for my mother and younger siblings. Expected to educate myself through distancelearning courses with no parental direction and with so many responsibilities, I lacked the credits to complete even my sophomore year. I did something crazy, I took the General Education Development test and entered college early. I had finished my high school biology and chemistry courses so I was able to start off college in freshman science courses.

This paragraph is one that just tells me what she did. She took the GED and started college early. This information doesn't tell me why she wants to be a physician, so it can be cut.

I dreamed about going to medical school, but I lacked guidance and support, and I was ignorant about the path to medical school. I knew it was expensive and I believed it was beyond my reach as my transition to adulthood proved challenging in unique ways. I left home as soon as I could because I was expected to maintain the same responsibilities that had held me back in high school. I had saved all my Alaska Permanent Fund dividends in a college fund, but my mother had spent it, and I had bad credit because she had used my identity. I received no support from my father. During these years, my mother overdosed several times. The difficulty of this period is reflected my early transcripts.

This is a very long red flag paragraph which ultimately tells me a lot of information that I don't really need to know. While the student had a lot of obstacles to overcome, the list here can be seen as placing blame. When you have obstacles, you have to own up to them. If you have a hard time owning up to them, don't place blame on others. Just leave it out of your personal statement. She could have easily put this in one sentence stating that, due to her mother's addiction, she struggled early academically.

After a year of typical courses for a biology major, I learned about the medical lab technology program. Only 2 years long, I would learn about blood cells, microbiology, the physiology of the organs. It was a perfect fit for me. I studied what I was deeply interested in and then I worked in hospital labs. Most importantly, I was able to better support myself, and escape from the long dark Alaskan winters.

Here the personal statement transitions to more of a timeline. This paragraph can easily be cut without losing much. It doesn't tell me anything about why medicine.

I planned to continue my education and I spent a semester studying nursing after making the move to the lower 48. However, life intervened and I made the decision to stay home when I had my first child, and our family quickly grew. Motherhood has been the hardest job I have ever had. I've had to constantly adapt to new circumstances and put the needs of others before my own. Like a doctor, a mother works long hours, is always on call and must carefully observe her charges to determine what is amiss when they are unable to communicate. A mother must constantly learn new things as her children are everchanging, and she must judiciously seek out evidence-based advice in a world full of opinions. When faced with a difficult task, I tell myself, if I have raised 5 kids, I can do anything.

> *Here is more backstory which doesn't tell me anything about why medicine. It helps explain who the student is, but I need to know why. The student needs to move on at this point. Right now, it seems like the student has life intervening at every step of the way, and I worry if the same thing will happen if she is admitted to medical school.*

With the kids in school, I found myself drawn once again to a career in the medical field. I jumped into a semester of difficult premed classes at the community college and kept up with my much younger classmates. I then considered following a more financially practical path and took a semester of nursing prerequisites, but I found myself bored and unchallenged by those classes. I hungered for the hard sciences and a deeper understanding of biology, so I transferred into the Molecular and Cellular Biology program at the University of Illinois and set my sites on medical school. Although I am unlike any of my classmates, I feel like I am right where I'm supposed to be.

> *This paragraph is still just giving me a timeline of events. It also includes a statement—"I found myself drawn once again to a career in the medical field"—that makes me ask "Why?" At this point, I'm still not sure why the student wants to be a physician. A lot of kids have parents who struggle with addiction. Not all of them go on to become physicians.*

Medical school would allow me to combine my love of learning with a career that would allow me to directly impact the lives of others. While I am entering this path later than most, with the love and support of my family and with so many life experiences behind me, I'm more prepared now than any other time in my life to embark on the path to becoming a physician.

> *Be careful with generic statements about* **why medicine.** *This student said medical school would "combine my love of learning with a career that would allow me to directly impact the lives of others." This statement is not specific to medicine. There are thousands of careers that would allow this student to learn and impact others.*

CP FIRST DRAFT

There were six beady-eyed students staring up at me with another one wandering around the room. Seven first graders were eagerly waiting for me to begin their first music lesson of the year. Unbeknownst to them, I was frozen in place filled to the brim with dread. Ever since I was ten years old, I dreamed of this exact moment. The moment I would start to build rapport and respect with students whom I would provide a safe haven of self-expression and creativity through music. And yet, here I was with my mind only ruminating on my huge mistake of career choice.

> *This is an interesting opening with great visuals. "Six beady-eyed students" is a great description of kids looking up at you. I'm left intrigued and wondering why this was a huge mistake. It makes me want to keep reading, which is good.*

Music meant the world to me ever since I held a clarinet in my hands. It was a whole new challenge that immediately became my passion. Music is an all-encompassing art form. It's not as simple as being proficient on a single instrument. As musicians, we have to simultaneously develop a deep understanding of a wide range of subjects from music theory, to history, to aural skills, to pedagogy. I was often overwhelmed by the diversity, but the challenge constantly drove me forward. I was, and always will be, drawn to music's technical complexities that challenged my body and mind. Performing breathing exercises, holding long tones, training your fingers all while mentally shaping phrases and planning musical expression is no easy feat. And yet, every ounce of frustration is worth the reward of achieving musical nirvana.

> *This paragraph is all about music. It doesn't tell me anything about the student's desire to become a physician. It's a story about music.*

The pinnacle of my musical career came during a Wind Ensemble performance of "Frozen Cathedral" by John Mackey. Mackey expertly placed intense dissonance to maximize the emotional power of the piece. In the last two minutes, the trombones have an incredibly powerful, dissonant entrance that soars over the band as a catharsis. This release was so immense tears just automatically streamed down my face and a lump in my throat made it impossible to keep my air flow strong. In these moments, it feels as it if I have reached the pinnacle of being human, as if the world has stopped spinning and everything has settled into its perfect place for just a fleeting moment. For twelve years of my life, I strove to create moments like this every day through music. That passion and drive is an essential part of who I am, and I believe that similar moments await in my career in medicine through interactions with my patients.

This paragraph continues like the previous one. It's a story about the student's music career with a quick "this is what my doctor life will be like" statement at the end. Remember previously when I mentioned that you should avoid tying your experiences in with being a physician? You don't know what medicine is like. You don't know what being a physician truly means until you become one.

Medicine itself is an art similar to music once you replace the technique of scales with the foundation of basic sciences and standard practices. Both rely on immense dedication to their foundation in order to create and navigate complex human emotions and situations to the ultimate improvement of lives. In music, each performance will be an entirely different experience just as each patient is unique. Music was not the perfect fit for my strengths and weaknesses. My brain is far too mathematically and rigid in order to hear the subtle differences in a symphony or to ever perform without sheet music. Medicine on the other hand will provide me the foundation, the standard practices, the format for me to then uniquely and creatively help each of my patients in immensely rewarding situations.

This whole paragraph is tying music to medicine. It doesn't need to be here. It doesn't give me any insight into why. *"Why do you want to be a physician?" is* the *question that you have to answer. That is not being done here.*

From the beginning of my musical career, I always knew performing was not for me. I was always more enthralled with the idea of teaching. I feel it is my duty to help those around me also understand and flourish in subject areas. I am not creative enough to develop unique, engaging lesson plans for a music class but in smaller settings, I flourish. As an organic chemistry teaching assistant, I am lucky enough to have miraculous moments each week with students. In one recitation, there was a particularly challenging question with an epoxide. One of my students was particularly defeated in the beginning of the recitation period; she was stressed out, closed off, and clearly frustrated. She had already given up to protect herself from potential failure. Naturally, I was determined to reverse her whole outlook. For the next twenty minutes, I slowly but steadily lead her group through the mechanism of the epoxide reaction using almost exclusively questions to build up their understanding. Before they knew it, they didn't just understand the single question but had a renewed sense of confidence with epoxides and themselves. I never gave up, I never passed them off to another teaching assistant. We did all preserved and walked out of that workshop on cloud nine as a result.

The student is informing me that she enjoys teaching. The question is: "Why not become a teacher?"

Being a physician is one of the most important teaching positions of all. I believe the cornerstone of my future responsibilities is to accurately and efficiently teach a patient and their family about their diagnosis and treatment options. Often patients are in extremely vulnerable situations they do not know how to navigate. They rely on doctors to provide them with the knowledge, power, and guiding light to make it through their future.

> *How does the student know that being a physician is one of the most important teaching positions of all? This paragraph just explains more about what she thinks medicine is like. Thinking that you know what medicine is like does not mean you should be a physician.*

From music to medicine, my undergraduate education provided me with a unique and powerful skill set that will both guide and enrich my personal path to becoming a physician. Medicine is a practice and an art, I can't wait to combine my artistic skills, discipline, and teaching abilities to create my future as a physician.

> *At the end, I'm left still asking why? Why does this student want to be a physician? What experiences has she had that have solidified this in her mind? What was the initial spark for her to decide to explore being a physician? This is a nice essay, but not a great personal statement. She went back to the drawing board. You can read her final draft next.*

CP FINAL DRAFT

I had just finished my first five-mile run. It took me an hour, but with every stride I was empowered by my body. Shortly following, I had to attend a college workshop featuring an electromyography biofeedback system meant to assess the tension in our bodies while playing bassoon. Peer after peer went with identical results: too much tension in their upper bodies. Despite the adrenaline in my system, my EMG was nearly flat. While I was not a master bassoon player, I did have an additional variable in my lifestyle: regularly working out. For the first time, my hours spent across campus in the gym had given me a clear advantage over my peers.

> *This is an interesting opening which gives me a glimpse at an unusual extracurricular—playing the bassoon. I'm intrigued and will read on. It doesn't tell me anything about medicine yet, but that's okay for now.*

With my new insight into the musical advantages of being in shape, I slowly watched two groups of music students emerge. One being my peers, who rarely suffered from any performance related pains, and everyone else. The latest wrist splints and neck straps were becoming increasingly popular among those unconcerned with their overall wellness. It dawned on me that as musicians, we rely on our small muscles for our technique and embouchure as much as a running back relies on his quadriceps. And yet, not a single credit hour was offered for us to learn about optimizing our physical wellness for a lifelong pursuit of performance.

> *I'm still wondering where this is taking me. I start to see some interest and intrigue around wellness, but I'm still questioning why this is important. This probably could have been cut to jump straight into the next paragraph.*

I immediately immersed myself in the field of musician's wellness. The more I researched, the more I felt at home with the topic. When I stumbled across the Performing Arts Medicine Association, my jaw dropped and a thought instantly took over my mind. Throughout my life I had aspirations of becoming a doctor. Medicine was an alternative path that I often daydreamt about, wondering how far I could push my love for science over music. Suddenly, medicine could become an option not solely driven by a what if, but powered by my lifelong passion for music.

Music transforms the human condition. While listening to music, people are often transported to an alternative emotional reality. For just a fleeting moment, it feels as it if I have reached the pinnacle of being human, as if the world has stopped spinning and everything has settled into its perfect place.

Now we're getting to the core of what the personal statement is about— **why medicine.** *The student wrote, "throughout my life I had aspirations of becoming a doctor." Why? These types of statements will always leave me asking why. You have to expand on a very generic statement like that. We're at the "seed" though. Now let's see where the student takes us to show how she "watered the seed."*

Outdoorsman hike, paddlers kayak, athletes play, and musicians perform in order to experience that same euphoria. I was disheartened to know that musicians could lose their own ability to perform due to performance-related injuries and in the process lose the ability to share this magic with others.

This is a very generic paragraph which has already been discussed previously. It could have been cut.

Reason speaks of a meaningful connection between music to medicine, but would medicine end up to be all I dreamed up? I soon found out one day at The Children's Medical Center while I was shadowing a pediatric oncology fellow. It was day two and I already knew the drill. Show up in the morning, find a comfy chair, and get ready for a couple hours of rounds. The day's discussion proceeded similarly to the previous when then the mood unexpectedly shifted: the gastrointestinal team had arrived.

The student is now trying to show us her experience with patients and the hospital setting. I'm a little confused by the statement "it was day two and I already knew the drill." It almost sounds like she was bored. She was bored until the gastrointestinal team showed up. In fact, an earlier draft mentioned how she struggled to keep her eyes open. Even with that removed, it still reads the same way. Be careful with potentially negative statements. The last thing you want me to think is that you're already bored with medicine.

There was an oncology patient that desperately needed an endoscopy. However, the GI team was convinced the patient would perforate. Both teams suddenly turned into gladiators and nothing else mattered. For the next hour, both teams methodically compared each other's plans. Neither team was right nor wrong. Yet, it was clear that the intensity in the room purely stemmed from passion for the patient's health. At this moment, medicine suddenly emerged as art. The passion and dedication radiating from each team sealed the deal that medicine was my perfect path to continue making both physical and emotional impacts on people's lives.

Here, I finally see what solidified the desire to become a physician for the student. It's interesting that the student writes about physicians having a debate as the reason that made her certain though. In a perfect world, I would have liked to see that the actual care for that patient is what is driving her.

As a medical assistant in a pulmonology practice, I often get the honor of making patients inhale and exhale as hard and as quickly as possible during spirometry testing. For weeks, I felt so guilty while conducting spirometry. I hated to be the face of a unpleasant and exhausting test; however, one day I realized that it is in these small moments when the humanity of medicine emerges. As a premed student, meaningful patient experience seems so far away, and yet here it was right under my nose. From that day forward, I brought in as much energy and enthusiasm into each test I conducted. I strive to be their personal cheerleader! Immediately, I noticed the positive effect this change had on both our moods and their performance! It is our responsibility as physicians to be the beacon of hope in even the most grueling situations.

> *This is a good story of a patient interaction and a realization that the student had that helped her enjoy the interaction more. What stands out, however, is that there are now two instances, one above, in which the student sounds bored during rounds, and this one, in which she was not having fun until she brought more energy and enthusiasm into the experience.*

Just as musicians combine technique, pedagogy, and expression, doctor's combine science, humanity, and collaboration to guide patients through some of life's biggest challenges. When I was ten years old, music changed my life. It provided me with a passion that I could share with others. With each and every medical experience, I have come to realize that there is an infinite number of ways to share my passion with patients across all specialties. Whether my patients are musicians, accountants, or grandparents, I will be able to make a positive impact on their lives through my medical practice. I have come to know medicine as a creative practice and art form. I look forward to applying my artistic skill and focused discipline towards a future as a physician.

> *This is a decent conclusion that wraps it all together. I wouldn't have suggested the tie-in with music. It's an example of the student trying to keep the theme of music going throughout the personal statement and wrapping it up with a neat little bow. It's not necessary, and more often than not it's just a waste of space. It works well enough in this personal statement. But, I would add: Can you think bigger? What do you want to accomplish as a physician? Here, she mentions using her "artistic skill" and "discipline" in the future. What will that accomplish? Try thinking bigger.*

JD FIRST DRAFT

Although I currently enjoy a successful, stable career as a programmer and computer engineer, I have chosen to pursue medicine due to a calling to assist people in a more meaningful and fulfilling way. The genesis for this decision came about with both a realization that I want more fulfillment in my life, and the self-discovery that in my leisure time, I find myself excitedly reading medical news articles instead of programming-related articles. I reflected on my willingness to watch my own surgical procedures performed with local anesthetic. In 2011, I had already begun my journey to change my life and career to one of service to others. It was during this time that I watched the catastrophic results of the explosion of a chemical plant in Jacksonville, Florida. I found myself feeling humble, yet hopeful with the anticipation that in a few years, I would be running toward the scene to be of service to those in need, rather than simply sitting idly by watching the news, feeling helpless.

Let's break this down a little bit. The first sentence tells me the student is a nontrad and wants to help people in a more meaningful and fulfilling way. Does this mean he should be a physician? Not at all. Helping people is not specific to medicine. Reading medical news articles doesn't mean you should be a physician either. The paragraph doesn't do what it's intended to do: give me a reason why.

Growing up, I was raised by a mother and father who did not have much, but still gave their time and efforts serving on the volunteer fire department and volunteer emergency medical service teams. During the summers, I would help my father in his side lawn-maintenance business. I remember seeing smoke billow up from the horizon. My father and I would stop work, and get in the truck. We headed to the fire to help the community and the owners of the unfortunate place that had caught fire. I remember my mother spending her evenings learning Spanish medical terms to help her perform as a volunteer EMT. This sacrifice, this call-to-duty, was something I have discovered I want to be in my life.

> *This is a good paragraph illuminating the student's upbringing. Two parents who gave to others through serving in EMS roles raised him. This type of earlier exposure can be a powerful draw to entering healthcare, yet it's not really mentioned as a draw, just as a "call-to-duty". A call-to-duty can be serving in the military, working in local politics, or something else, other than being a physician. The takeaway needs to change to reflect the patient care associated with being a physician, not just a call-to-duty.*

As a volunteer in the hospital, I was able to push or walk with patients either to their rooms or to a car for pick up. I was able to talk with the patients and help care for them, whether getting a warmed blanket, or listening to them express any concerns they were having. I loved being a part of the team that cared for these patients in some of their most vulnerable experiences in their lives. It was humbling to consider my role in taking the patient from a moment of sickness or pain, to being able to return to their home. Thinking about the physician's role in leading the effort to help the patient get to this better state of health only reinforced my resolve.

> *This is a great example of a* telling *paragraph. "I was able to push," "I was able to talk," "It was humbling." This could have been much more effective with a story of a patient interaction.*

In the emergency department, I remember one night a person came to the desk saying her husband was having chest pains in the car. I grabbed a wheelchair and quickly went to the car. I helped him get in the car and brought him straight to a room for diagnosis and care by the trained staff members. While being proud to provide a part of the service to this patient, I wanted to be able to help in a more important role.

Here's the story. This could have been worked into the previous paragraph to highlight what he was discussing.

In one of my shadowing experiences, the surgeon allowed me to scrub in to assist in minor roles during a cesarean section. Moments before making the first incision, he leans over to me and asks if I am okay around blood. I assure him I am, and he begins. He asks me to hold the retractor during the procedure and I will always remember the surprising wave of amniotic fluid that covered my hand and wrist when the sac was broken. This exciting event was quickly outdone by the emergence of new life that was rushed to the mother's arms, bringing back memories of being present for my own children's births.

Be careful with tense. The previous paragraph used past tense—
"grabbed" and "brought." This paragraph is in present tense—
"he asks" and "he leans." Keep the tense consistent.
Past tense is usually the best. What is the takeaway of this experience?
How does it lead to wanting to be a physician?

The culmination of these thoughts, experiences, and events have only reinforced my desire to change my life and seek one where I can not only be a part of, but lead a team of medical staff members in the care of patients in the health of their lives.

What is the goal for the future? Being part of, and leading, a team of medical staff members is great, but what else? Think bigger. You can read his final draft on the next page.

JD FINAL DRAFT

Watching the smoke rising from the catastrophic explosion at a chemical plant in Jacksonville, Florida, I felt helpless. I was sitting watching on the news, when what I really wanted to be doing was running toward the scene to help those in need. I knew at this moment that I had made the right decision three years ago to begin on my path to medical school.

> *This is a great visual. It makes me picture the smoke rising, and it immediately conveys the student's mindset.*

Although I currently enjoy a successful, stable career as a programmer and computer engineer, I have chosen to pursue medicine due to a calling to play a more active role in my community. The decision for this change came about with both a realization that I have wanted more fulfillment in my life, and the self-discovery of remembering the role models in my life doing what they could to better their community in volunteer emergency services. This passion has always been with me. At the end of my high school education, I was at the crossroads of considering a major for college. I strongly considered medicine, but I held myself back and steered myself away from this dream. I blocked myself and my dreams with a self-imposed doubt that my small-school education had prepared me for success at the college level, and I could not imagine myself able to shoulder the immense responsibility of patients' health and more so their lives.

> *This is an excellent explanation of being a nontraditional student and explaining why, if he had these passions "always," he didn't pursue them earlier. This immediately removes any questions I may have asked during an interview.*

Growing up, I was raised by a mother and father who did not have much, but still gave their time and efforts serving on the volunteer fire department and volunteer emergency medical service teams. In the summertime, I would help my father in his lawn-maintenance business. I remember one day seeing smoke billow up from the horizon. My father and I stopped work, and got in the truck. We headed directly to the residence that had caught fire to help put it out. It was a service to the community to keep the fire from spreading to the surrounding, tall, dry brush and to the owner of the unfortunate place that had caught fire. I remember my mother spending her evenings learning Spanish medical terms to help her perform as a volunteer EMT. I talked to her about why she was taking these classes and her response embodied her devotion to helping others and taking on the responsibility to help. This sacrifice, this call-to-duty, is something that has been missing in my life and I do not want its absence anymore. I am finally ready to pursue it.

> *This story is carried forward from the previous draft. The takeaway is the same—the "call-to-duty." It could be a stronger, with a more direct line to healthcare and being a physician, but it's a start.*

Volunteering in the emergency department, there was one night a person came to the front desk saying her husband was having chest pains in the car. I grabbed a wheelchair and quickly went to the car. I helped him get in the car and brought him straight to a room for diagnosis and care by the trained staff members. While being proud to provide a part of the service to this patient, I wanted to be able to help in a more important role.

> *The takeaway here is a very common sentiment that students have: "I wanted to be able to help in a more important role." This is incredibly common, especially for students coming from other healthcare fields like nursing or being a physician assistant.*

While shadowing a trauma physician, there was a case where an eighteen-year-old patient had just had an automobile accident, losing both of his legs. Before entering the room, the physician not only spoke of the physical implications with the patient, but also the emotional trauma the patient was going through, and how to helping the patient emotionally deal with this major life change was something the doctor was addressing. It was a moving moment to understand the roles the physicians take on in such important and life-changing moments of patient's lives.

> *This is a good patient encounter that could have been made a little more effective with a better takeaway. The takeaway here is an understanding of what physicians do. Just because you* think *you understand what a physician does, doesn't mean you should become one. You have to dig a little deeper.*

In another of my shadowing experiences, the surgeon allowed me to scrub in to assist in minor roles during a Cesarean section. Moments before making the first incision, he leaned over to me and asked if I am okay around blood. I assured him I am, and he began. He asked me to hold the retractor during the procedure. I will always remember the surprising wave of amniotic fluid that covered my hand and wrist when the amniotic sac was broken. This exciting event was quickly outdone by the emergence of new life that was rushed to the mother's arms. Not only was I not uncomfortable with the blood and bodily fluids, I knew in my heart that this is what I want to do in my life.

> *Notice that this paragraph has switched to past tense. There are some great descriptions like the "wave of amniotic fluid." There is a strong takeaway here that brings it all together .*

One moment that has stuck with me ten years later is the night I was sitting in the waiting room with family after my wife's grandfather passed away of a heart attack. The doctor entered the room and sat down. He compassionately, but honestly spoke with my wife's grandmother to tell her the sad news. I play back this moment in my head often. This part of the profession must never get easy, but I believe it is an important and noble role in the world. It is a calling that I feel the need and desire to fulfill so that I can give back to the world.

> *This is another quick story from a personal experience with a good takeaway.*

The culmination of these thoughts, experiences, and events have only reinforced my desire to change my life and seek one where I can not only be a part of, but lead a team of medical staff members in the care of patients in the health of their lives. Although I regret not pursuing this path earlier, I am certain that the life I have led and the experiences I have had to this point will make me a better physician.

> *This has a similar ending to the last paragraph; a brief reflection on not pursuing this path earlier. It could have been more ambitious, with more wide-ranging ideas regarding what he hopes to accomplish as a physician, but the added piece of reflection is nice.*
> *This student is attending an allopathic medical school in Texas.*

MC FIRST DRAFT

At the time of our meeting, Jane was a middle age woman who had struggled with weight for most of her adult life. Recently told by her doctor that she was pre-diabetic, Jane had finally found the impetus to seek out ways to improve her health. Diabetes was a disease that ran in Jane's family and she wanted to ensure that she would not incur the same fate. As a trainer, I was aware that lifestyle played a significant role in managing diabetes although I was unfamiliar with the underlying disease process. I was confident, however, that with my help she could improve her health and reduce her risk of developing diabetes.

At the start of this statement, the student describes being a personal trainer, which indicates to me that he is possibly a nontraditional student. I want to learn a little more.

Diabetes also runs in my family; for 2 years while in elementary school I remember living with my grandparents as we relocated back to New York from military life in California. Every morning before school, I would eat breakfast with my grandmother who also suffered from diabetes. I would mix and match cereals but she always had the same thing, special K cereal and skim milk. It was a stringent protocol that I was told she needed to follow in order to control her illness. Despite these efforts, as I grew older my grandmother's diabetes continued to worsen and was followed by a number of health problems resulting in coronary bypass surgery and eventually a massive stroke which left her physically limited.

This is some backstory of a possible "seed" that was planted, but I'm not sure because the student doesn't tell me why the information in this paragraph is important.

As a personal trainer I worked with a number of clients who, like Jane, were looking to me to improve their health. Many brought with them an implicit fear that maintaining their current lifestyle risked the inevitable onset of chronic disease. If I was going to expand my clientele, it was necessary that I be able to communicate the role of proper exercise and nutrition on managing chronic disease. This meant that I would need to become more fluent in the science and medicine of common chronic diseases such as diabetes.

We're headed back into the possible seed with the student now writing about needing to learn more about diabetes.
We're circling around without getting anywhere.

The more I learned the more I came to understand the very real limitations of my scope of knowledge. Complicating matters further, the available evidence seemed to conflict regarding the efficacy of different lifestyle interventions. The field of nutrition continues to be in the midst of an internal debate about the role of certain foods in promoting health. My research did little to help me more clearly articulate the benefit of certain interventions; rather it left me with more questions than answers. I felt compelled to understand the disease process at a deeper level rather than just a cursory review of the facts. After almost a year I had to come to a realization that to remain in this role would limit my expanding intellectual curiosity into these topics and ultimately limit my ability to intervene on others behalf.

We're still circling around and haven't learned much more about any reasons why this student is applying to medical school.
You need to try to be concise and get the message across quickly.
Remember, you don't have a lot of characters with which to work.

In college I worked weekends in a hospital near my home and during many evenings had found myself in the ER delivering supplies to the nursing staff. This is where I first encountered medical scribes, as they worked alongside ER physicians feverishly taking down notes. My time as a trainer had left me searching to fill an intellectual void but it had convinced me that any future role I pursued should be people-centered. The draw to medicine was starting to take hold and working as a medical scribe offered the best opportunity to learn the intimate details of life as a physician.

> *There is a little "why not personal training" in this paragraph. The student mentions why he didn't like being a trainer—due to an "intellectual void." Focus on* why *medicine, not* why not *your previous career/job.*

The emergency room allowed me to experience medicine in all of its vagaries. My mother has been an ER nurse for most of her life and spent several years in trauma so I was not ignorant of the ER's reputation for high-stress heroics. What most surprised me, however, was the number of patients who use the ER due to a lack of access to adequate medical care. As a result, many of the patients who I see regularly in the ED suffer from complications due to the poor management of their chronic illnesses. This experience has further strengthened my desire to become a physician so that I will possess the skills necessary to treat acute illness but also use my platform to promote preventive care.

> *Here we finally start seeing some* why *medicine. This student wants to promote preventive medicine. This is the first time he's mentioned his extensive exposure to medicine due to his mom being a nurse. He could have brought this up earlier. This paragraph could have been focused better with a story.*

I was admittedly reluctant following my undergraduate experience to put the full weight of my expectations into pursuing medicine. However, each day at work I am reminded why the path to becoming a physician is fraught with challenges. In the years since leaving college, I have had the opportunity to explore interests and reflect on my prior academic difficulties...

The first draft ends without a conclusion because, at the time, the student was struggling to come up with one. It can be hard, if you don't have great stories and thoughts for the rest of your essay, to succinctly wrap everything up for an ending. I'm still left wondering why medicine. I don't know why this student wants to be a doctor. You can't leave me still questioning why. You can read his final draft next.

MC FINAL DRAFT

At the time of our meeting, Jane was a middle age woman who had struggled with weight for most of her adult life. Recently told by her doctor that she was pre-diabetic, Jane had finally found the impetus to seek out ways to improve her health. Diabetes was a disease that ran in Jane's family and she wanted to ensure that she would not incur the same fate. As a trainer, I was aware that lifestyle played a significant role in managing diabetes although I was unfamiliar with the underlying disease process. I was confident, however, that with my help she could improve her health and reduce her risk of developing diabetes.

This is the same start to the first draft. Nothing needed to be changed.

As a personal trainer I worked with a number of clients who, like Jane, were looking to me to improve their health. Many brought with them an implicit fear that maintaining their current lifestyle risked the inevitable onset of chronic disease. If I was going to expand my clientele, it was necessary that I be able to communicate the role of proper exercise and nutrition on managing chronic disease. This meant that I would need to become more fluent in the science and medicine of common chronic diseases such as diabetes.

Can you see how the student has removed the discussion about his family? It added a lot of characters to the personal statement without adding any insight. We're being told that something needed to change in the student's life. In his previous draft, he circled around this point for too long; here he is more direct.

An internal conflict arose as I came to understand the limitations of my scope of knowledge. My research into different lifestyle interventions had done little to help me more clearly articulate their benefits to my clients; rather it left me with more questions than answers. I felt compelled to understand the disease process at a deeper level rather than just a cursory review of the facts. It became apparent that while exercise and nutrition can be the foundations of maintaining good health, many of my clients were dealing with health problems that required a far more intensive understanding of the human body. I desired to pursue a career that would not limit my sphere of influence within the narrow confines of exercise and nutrition. I also knew the management of the chronic conditions that so fascinated me were in the purview of medicine. Despite this realization, I remained hesitant about a future career in medicine but knew this was a path I needed to explore more deeply.

This paragraph tells us exactly what the student was thinking when he decided to pursue exploring more about medicine.

In college, I worked in a hospital near my home and this is where I first encountered medical scribes in the ER. Working as a scribe offered an opportunity to work closely with physicians so I could see if this was a future I wanted to pursue. As a scribe, what had the greatest impact on me was the ability of ER physicians to remain calm and centered in the face of life-threatening situations. I recall one particularly busy night when the ER attending was managing several critical patients with several more patients waiting to be seen. We found ourselves in the room of a woman in her 50's who had developed a rapid heart rate suddenly after dinner and on arrival was nearing 200 beats per minute. The ER physician explained that she was in SVT and he would be administering a medication that could break the abnormally high rhythm. In the room, the woman was seated on the stretcher visibly anxious and fearful with her nervous husband beside her. The ER physician, despite the responsibility of a busy department and other critical patients, remained relaxed and maintained his focus on his patient. I watched as he eased her fear by sitting at the edge of the stretcher, holding her hand and cracking jokes while involving the husband in conversation to distract from the nurse readying to deliver the bolus of medication.

This is a good showing *paragraph that describes a patient encounter. A good takeaway seems to be missing, but it's actually at the start of the next paragraph.*

It is moments like these that serve as a continual reminder of why I chose to pursue a career in medicine. As an immature undergraduate lacking a clear vision for the future, I struggled academically to perform to the level of my ability. When I decided to begin preparing for the MCAT 3 years ago and return to academia, there was a shift in how I approached my studies. During the process, when met with moments of struggle, I could draw upon my past experiences as inspiration. With this clarity of mind I was able to achieve a level of performance that better reflected my academic potential.

This is a red flag statement. The student is telling me that there are some bad grades on his transcript, and he provides a reason for them. This is good, but it probably could have been a little shorter to make more room for more about why medicine.

Having been on the periphery of the physician-patient relationship for several years, I look into the future with great anticipation as I imagine one day caring for my own patients. I am reminded of Jane and other clients who came to me looking for ways to improve their health. The inability to do so started me on this journey and it remains my hope that as a physician those answers will be within my grasp.

This is a good conclusion which uses the story of his personal training client, Jane, and how she ultimately led to his desire to become a physician. This ending continues the general trend in conclusions that could be a little more expansive in terms of future goals to accomplish as a physician. This student is attending an osteopathic medical school in the Midwest.

KS EARLY DRAFT

When I was younger, I was drawn to medicine by a love of learning and problem-solving. As an adult and through my experiences in the military, I now know my motivation is derived from a deep-rooted love of service. Additionally, I believe in order to have an opportunity to succeed in employment and education, all humans require a baseline level of health. My goal has become to serve my community by providing this opportunity. I believe the best way to meet this goal is as a physician.

> *I've come to call this a "mission statement" opening.*
> *Students commonly include these at the start of their personal*
> *statements. They're not needed. They take up valuable space that you*
> *could be using to show me who you are.*

In middle and high school I was fortunate and watched surgeries over the summers. I was in awe of the processes which allow the human body to function and was drawn to medicine. When I was fourteen, I discovered my purpose. With the invasion of Iraq in 2003, my mother, an Army physician, had her first deployment when I was thirteen. Parents, siblings, and spouses were deployed, lost, and sometimes returned deeply changed. I was fortunate my mother returned home whole and largely the woman I remember. Sometime after my mother's return, a memorial was written in the local newspaper celebrating soldiers who sacrificed their lives. I vividly remember my mother pointing to the faces of the soldiers she couldn't save. I could tell the loss was overwhelming, but I also knew that for each face on that page, she and her team saved hundreds of others. I changed in that moment, I knew I wanted to serve those who chose to devote their lives to freedom. Over time this purpose has morphed to include my greater community, military and civilian.

The student starts off by telling us a lot of great information. First, she is the daughter of a physician. This helps me understand who the student is. It doesn't necessarily help the student, but as a reader, it gives me a little more understanding. Second, it almost gives me her "seed." Her mom was a military physician, and now the student says she wants to "serve" those who devote their lives to freedom. Serving can mean many things. This paragraph could be shorter. There are a lot of extra details that don't add anything to the personal statement.

In high school, my mom deployed two more times. Each time she returned, she told me how the improved technology, training, and medical transport resulted in fewer fatalities, even given the same injuries. I remained fascinated and committed. To accomplish part of my goal, I pursued military service at the Academy.

In the previous paragraph, the student said she wanted to serve. She is continuing that thinking by writing about going to the Academy.

I initially declared my major as Biology, following the premed track, but I grew bored memorizing facts and became more interested in assessing and solving problems. During this time I also experienced a personal tragedy, lost much of my motivation to succeed, and strongly considered leaving the Academy. I maintained, although less clearly, my goal of being a physician. The Academy prepares students to serve, my ultimate goal. I eventually decided to stay.

Here is some negativity that can be thrown out. The student "grew bored." Is she going to grow bored during medical school classes too? It's a lot of memorizing as well. She also brings up a potential red flag in her transcripts regarding a personal tragedy. I'm not sure what she means by "less clearly." Is she questioning becoming a physician?

The Academy didn't have a path that directly merged health and engineering, my two interests, but I found the applications of environmental engineering intriguing. I learned how health is intricately tied to the environment and influences the likelihood of developing cancer, education outcomes, the ability to move out of poverty, and so much more. I was able to integrate chemical and biological processes into problem-solving with a focus of minimizing negative health outcomes.

> *The student is describing merging health and engineering, but hasn't yet told us she wants to be a physician. I can assume that, since this is a personal statement for the medical school application, but it could be made a little more obvious. I'm not sure what this paragraph is telling me. I don't think it's adding anything at this point.*

I shifted over the next year between a few different paths. I thought maybe I could serve as an Explosive Ordinance Disposal officer, preventing the numerous blast injuries instead of treating them after they occurred, or I could facilitate combatant care by flying medical evacuation aircraft. But, I always remembered that day with my mom and the newspaper.

> *This is a good paragraph about reflection, but ultimately it doesn't add much to her story. It's almost like a mini résumé.*

During my junior year I was selected for pilot training. I struggled with the selection. I knew there was a chance I would be selected to fly an aircraft with a primary mission of killing people instead of saving them. I felt it would be wrong for me. Instead, I applied to be a Bioenvironmental Engineer which focuses on preventative health actions. I struggled during my first two years at the Academy, but my performance and research during the last two years resulted in my selection in the preventative healthcareer field as well as an graduate school position.

> *Here we're into full résumé mode. The student has now switched from the storytelling she did at the beginning with her mom, to giving me a timeline of what was going on in her life.*

After graduate school, I spent three years working in preventative health at the military base. It was there my passion for medicine returned. I led teams that interfaced between the medical facility and the work centers we supported. We assessed hazards and developed risk profiles used by commanders to make decisions. We worked closely with many physicians to understand and screen vulnerable populations. We designed solutions to minimize acute and chronic occupational health risks, but were also constantly on call for any biological, chemical, radiological, or nuclear emergency. We were also called when there was an overexposure, aircraft mishap, or unexplained health outcome.

> *This paragraph is showing some uniqueness in the student's path, though it could be improved with some more showing statements. It also doesn't tell me specifically why this added to her wanting to be a physician. I could argue that if she liked doing this, why not continue it?*

I also had to grapple with many workers who didn't want to comply, they didn't want to wear a respirator or work with a cumbersome ventilation system. They just wanted to do their job without extra burden. This was when I truly understood the deep relationship between medicine and education. Once workers understood the impact of daily practices on their health and that of their families, they welcomed our recommendations.

> *Similar to the last paragraph, how did coming to the conclusion that education is important further the student's desire to be a physician?*

I currently serve as an Environmental Engineering Instructor back at the Academy, which I believe has prepared me more than any other experience. My most challenging responsibility is to communicate complex ideas effectively to my students. I've learned that my knowledge, while important, isn't enough. I have to step back from "this is the knowledge" to first assess what preconceived notions each student brings, how they learn, how they process, and how they express comprehension. I think this understanding of how people learn is integral to providing effective healthcare.

> *This student falls into the trap of discussing what she believes is "integral to providing effective healthcare." Remember, you don't have to tell me why you're going to be a good doctor, or that you understand what being a doctor is all about. I just want to know* why.

I am grateful I did not attend medical school immediately following my undergraduate degree. My experiences as an adult and in the military have sharpened my understanding of what I want to do – serve my community by providing education-based healthcare. When I graduated, I looked at a problem and generated a solution. Now, I am able to step back and form a solution with an awareness and understanding of the problem, goals, and resulting impacts. As a physician, I'll be able look at the whole person instead of just the symptoms; to see the forest instead of just the trees.

At the end of reading this draft, I'm still left with the question of why. What started with some promise, quickly turned into a résumé and discussion of the skills she thinks she has that will make her a good physician. You don't need to do this. Write about your why. Write about your personal story. You can read her final draft on the next page.

KS FINAL DRAFT

In middle and high school I was fortunate to watch surgeries with my mom over the summers. The experiences made me curious about the complexity of human systems, and I felt a desire to pursue medicine. When I was fourteen, my desire was coupled with purpose. My mother, a Army physician, had her first deployment as part of the invasion of Iraq in 2003. After her return, the local paper wrote a memorial commemorating the soldiers who sacrificed their lives. I vividly remember her pointing, one at a time, to the faces of the Marines she couldn't save. I could tell the loss was overwhelming, but I also knew that for each face on that page, she and her team saved hundreds of others. I changed in that moment–I knew I wanted to care for those who dedicated their lives to a higher purpose.

Here, the student starts very similarly to the draft on the previous pages. She does a good job of making her ideas very specific to medicine. She gives us her "seed." Her mom was a military physician, and now the student wants to care for patients the same way her mom did.

In high school my mom deployed two more times. Each time she returned, she shared how the improved technology, training, and accelerated medical transport resulted in fewer fatalities. These conversations conveyed medicine's hope of providing second chances for these young men and women to pursue their dreams. Through my service and long connection to the military community, I've also seen that for the severely sick or injured, their medical battles are often just beginning. The struggle to maintain quality of life, functional capability, and spirit takes place over time, often years. No matter the patient, military or civilian, I want to contribute to their fight as a physician.

> *Take a look at that last sentence. It's a strong takeaway.*
> *She's connected to the military community as a daughter of a soldier*
> *and she has the desire to serve, as her mother has.*

My grades dipped during my sophomore year of college, and I wasn't able to pursue medicine directly after graduation and commissioning. Still, I sought a health-related career in the military and was selected for preventive health. There my passion for medicine grew, and I decided to pursue my path to medical school. Working in preventive health, my teams and I worked closely with physicians to protect our military members. We assessed hazards and designed solutions to minimize acute and chronic health risks. The work, while engaging and important, wasn't enough. I always wanted to be involved from a different perspective. I wanted to understand and combat the underlying mechanisms making the patients ill. I wanted to be the one conducting the patient interviews. I wanted to be the one receiving them in the emergency room. I wanted to be the one following up. I wanted to be their physician.

> *Here, we're given more of who this student is. Her military career helps*
> *the student stand apart from others. This is how you add the "personal"*
> *into a personal statement. It's also tied to* **why medicine.** *She was*
> *working together with physicians, helping patients, but never in the role*
> *she wanted. The paragraph finishes with another strong takeaway.*

I was selected to run emergency preparedness exercises during the time Ebola emerged as a prominent international threat. I had two responsibilities: first, my preventive health teams prepared deploying service members to support the containment and treatment mission in Africa, and, second, I designed methods to test our medical facility's ability to contain and care for returning deployers. We designed an exercise, injects, and various decision trees. I researched the disease process, transmission, and isolation procedures, thriving on the opportunity to understand how different specialties and medical systems facilitated continuous and safe patient care. After directing simulations in isolation rooms, I was sure–I didn't want to be running the simulation; I wanted to be the one practicing medicine.

This paragraph is very similar to the last one. It continues to show the student in her role as a member of the military, on the periphery of medicine, but wanting to step into the role of a physician.

I have shadowed in multiple communities over the years. As I've seen the joy, love, loss, and hope in patients and their families, my purpose has broadened to serve both military and civilian communities. I believe every person deserves an opportunity to contribute and benefit society. Health is a central tenant of this opportunity and, once satisfied, provides a springboard for other positive outcomes. At a free clinic in Detroit, I noticed a common theme in the patients – they just wanted to keep going. Some wanted to keep working, others to keep learning or caring for their children, but their goals were generally derived from a loss of function. I vividly remember one patient, a construction worker, with a severe rash on his back so debilitating that his ability to work was limited. The physician prescribed an ointment and began reviewing the instructions, but paused and asked, "Do you have someone to help you apply the ointment?" A smile filled his face and he shared his family with us. It was amazing, in such a short interaction, the physician helped him return to health so he could live a better life, provide opportunities for his children, and continue to contribute to society.

The student does an interesting thing in this paragraph. She has initially focused on the military. This may turn off some public medical schools, whose job it is to train future physicians for their states. In this paragraph, she opens up and explains she may not be solely looking at military medicine. She also shows us an interaction with a patient she enjoyed and how it impacted her.

I am grateful I did not attend medical school immediately following my undergraduate degree. My experiences as an adult and in the military have sharpened my understanding of my goals. Like the physicians in Detroit, in the Ebola simulations, and like my mom, I want to serve and benefit my community through the pursuit of healthcare for all.

> *Here, the student ties everything together and gives a simple conclusion along with her goals.*
> *Similar to previous nontraditional personal statements, this student makes it a point to show her nontraditional side. It's what makes it personal. It's her story. She weaves medicine into her career in the military and effectively shows me why she is committed to this path.*

JuD FIRST DRAFT

Over the years, my medical interests helped me excel in the science track in high school to the point of becoming a certified first aid and CPR instructor. I knew that I wanted to be a physician. However, after high school, the stark reality of my family's humble status came to bear. I was compelled to find a job to support my family financially, tempering any hopes of going to college, or becoming a physician. However, with great determination, I was able to secure a one-year partial tuition scholarship, and in total opposition to my parents' wishes, I went to college.

> *What does this opening tell me? It doesn't tell me much, other than that the student excels in science and he knew he wanted to be a physician. This is the furthest from where you want to start a personal statement. Remember, the goal is for me to want to keep reading. This doesn't do it.*

With the pressure of being the first in my family to go to college, I had to choose a major that afforded me the shortest route to a secure job in order to provide financially for my family. A major in Computer Science provided the requisite personal academic challenge and fulfilled my family obligations. But the desire to enter the medical profession was not quenched.

> *Right now, we're diving into a résumé in essay form. This is a very common mistake students make.*

After financing my way through college, I resumed my familial duty of providing financially while working as a computer teacher and attending graduate school. My responsibilities expanded as I sent both my sister and sister-in-law to college, and supported my wife through graduate school. I tried to forget medicine but one memorable experience brought me face to face with my first love. As a computer programmer, I worked with dentists and scientists from State University and Software Company to create a head and neck anatomy encyclopedia software for dental students. This time I could not turn away, and fortunately, for the first time in my life I did not have to choose between family obligations and my passion for medicine.

> *This paragraph continues the theme of a résumé. We keep learning more about* what *the student has done, but we haven't learned* who *the student is or* why *he is doing these things.*

Questioning whether it was too late to pursue medicine, I decided to volunteer and shadow doctors in a variety of specialties. I began by shadowing a radiologist at the State University Medical Center and later volunteered in the Emergency Department of the County Regional Medical Center (CRMC) where I observed the high-intensity coordination of the team of doctors, nurses, ER techs and EMTs coalescing around the single aim of saving lives. I also shadowed a family medicine physician at his practices at the CRMC and the Family Care Center.

> *Again, more about* what *the student is doing. All of this is listed already in the extracurricular activity section.*

In addition, I shadowed five surgeries at the Ambulatory Surgical Center, observing pre- and post-operative consults with nurses, anesthesiologists, and surgeons. It was a remarkable opportunity to be allowed to stand close to an orthopedic surgeon as he provided me step-by-step explanations throughout the surgeries. With a greater desire for more patient-centric exposure, I began volunteering as a medical scribe at the New Free Clinic where I was able to do patient intake, counsel patients, scribe for doctors, shadow several minor surgeries, and train other doctors and nurses on how to use of the electronic health records system.

> *I think you can see the trend continuing here.*

Finally, my wife and I cofounded a free medical, dental, and mental health clinic called One Health. We were able to assemble a team of medical volunteers that provide services once per month and since we've opened our doors all appointment slots have been booked. We are grateful for the ability to give back to a community that desperately needs healthcare services.

> *Now, this is getting a little interesting. The student founded a free health clinic. He didn't volunteer at one. He founded it! That is interesting. Unfortunately, it's at the very end of the personal statement, and most readers are probably done reading by this point.*

These experiences validated my pursuit of medicine and removed all misgivings. I am now eager, if given the opportunity, to undertake this path of humble service of providing essential healthcare to others as a physician.

> *This personal statement draft is the perfect example of a resume in essay form. It doesn't tell me anything about* who *the student is, only that he has done most of the common extracurriculars that other premed students also do.*

JuD FINAL DRAFT

We stood outside, a mass of bodies sweating in the sweltering Florida sunshine. Around us were the gritty, low-income apartments and run-down single family homes that bracketed the parking lot where we gathered. The main door was decorated with a velveteen congratulatory red ribbon that signified the Chamber of Commerce was about to perform another ribbon cutting ceremony for a new business. This was our business, One Health, a free clinic in Tampa, Fl.

Remember the first draft. The one highlight was that the student founded a health clinic. We brought it to the front to highlight it. This is what is going to make him stand out.

It was an easy decision for my wife and I to dip into our finances as well as a reservoir of faith to bootstrap this operation: a free medical and dental clinic, fully staffed by volunteer providers who give their time and talent. In addition to work, school, and family, I was also busy cleaning clinic rooms, transporting medical and dental equipment, training volunteers, setting up the electronic medical records system, and chairing the clinic's board meetings. The unselfish and constant devotion with which my mom, a woman of little means, provided free midwifery services, family planning classes, and food and clothing to our community, has impressed upon me from a very young age to give to my community.

We get a little backstory to the clinic, and we also get our first glimpse into a possible "seed." His mom was a midwife. We didn't get that information last time. He also has a takeaway here, which is important, but could be more impactful. Right now, it's about giving to the community, but you can give back through any career.

I can't stop staring at the clinic's door. Doors have become a recurring theme in my life, and this clinic was just another in a series of entrances to opportunities that have shaped my life. Immediately, my mind was seamlessly transported to the humid living room of my parents' small home in Guyana. I stared at the forbidden door that held the mysteries of childbirth behind it. I heard my mother, a seasoned midwife, utter clipped instructions to laboring mothers. I contemplated on the importance of my mother's work in communities that lacked resources and access, where she provided midwifery services to mothers who otherwise could not afford it. My mom's respect for her patients, regardless of socio-economic status, has impressed upon me to be a caring medical provider to communities like ours.

We're getting great **showing** *statements. "Staring at the clinic's door." I can picture the student standing there, waiting to go in. We get an even deeper look at how his mom's midwife practice influenced him. The takeaway here is tied more closely to medicine, which is better.*

It was because of her that I joined the Pathfinder Club (a coed version of scouts) at age seven. I became energetically involved in weekly school lunch distributions, quarterly cleaning of senior citizens or disabled persons' homes, semi-annual visits to geriatric or pediatric hospital wards, semi-annual health fair and anti-drug marches, and a yearly penny drive to provide funds to needy and natural disaster victims. I became a Pathfinder counselor at age fifteen and the associate director at eighteen and thus for most of my life have been planning and executing these events, teaching Pathfinder classes, and most importantly modeling young lives to be responsible citizens. My burning desire to once again directly contribute to my community was satisfied as we, through this clinic, tackle a grossly underserved community serviced by only a few primary care providers.

The student gives me a glimpse at a formative experience from his upbringing. He's been giving back to the community since he was seven-years-old, and he wants to continue that; he brings this back to the clinic he founded.

As supporters strolled into the parking lot, the President of the Chamber called everyone to order, the ceremony ensued, and the ribbon was officially cut. A volunteer opened the door and ushered us inside. The previous week I walked through a door similar to this. That door stood ajar under a large sign proclaiming the location of the New Start Free Clinic in Tampa, FL. I am grateful to have helped to keep that door of opportunity open for others for almost two years. I have ushered in men who have not seen a doctor in years, women who chose their family's food and shelter over their medical care, and children who are used to translating complex medical information for their parents.

> *The student continues to highlight his biggest differentiator, the clinic. It not only shows that he is entrepreneurial, organized, a leader, etc., it also shows a strong commitment to healthcare.*

One day I held those doors open for a couple. The husband presented for a minor surgical procedure to remove a cyst from behind his right ear. But his blood pressure was elevated and the surgery was delayed. Since he was unaware of uncontrolled blood pressure at home, the physician decided to wait until his blood pressure stabilized. I sat with him and his wife and decided to talk with them to ease his anxiety in an effort to decrease his blood pressure. He conversed easily, as he bragged about his beautiful granddaughter and her love for mangoes. Moments became minutes, each one bringing him closer to normal blood pressure. I assisted the physician who performed the surgery, and I got to see the satisfied smile of yet another grateful patient. This encounter taught me to always put patient comfort first, listen attentively, and interact patiently regardless of my time commitment.

> *This is our first glimpse of a patient interaction, showing me some empathy and compassion from the student, without him explicitly saying that he is empathic or compassionate. The takeaway shows me what type of physician this student could be.*

I am carried along with the wave of onlookers viewing the clinic's equipment. I stop in the last patient room and look around thoughtfully reminiscing on how I've learnt to respond humbly to every patient's need as my mom did, greet every patient with a smile, regardless of working conditions, as a primary care physician I shadowed encouraged me, and never stop learning as an anesthesiologist mentor admonished me. Although not clinically involved with this clinic, I am hopeful, if given the opportunity, to be able to one day provide patient care to such a community. I usher the last of the well-wishers through the back door and thank them for coming. Then I stroll determinedly to the front door of the clinic and open it to welcome the waiting patients in.

> *"Think bigger" has been a common critique of the previous conclusions. Well, this one is pretty big. He's touring his facility and commenting on how he wants to provide care to a similar community. This is a very strong personal statement and the student received a lot of interview invites because of it.*
> *This student is attending an allopathic medical school in California.*

TJ FIRST DRAFT

I am engaged. And like my friends who are engaged, but in a much different way, I am elated. Engaged is a word a woman of my age, from a small town in rural Alabama, hears quite often. The pressure to be engaged is palpable. In fact, where I come from being unattached at age twenty-four is bordering on being considered an old maid. But I am not affianced like my schoolyard friends who are finding mates, becoming betrothed and ushering down the aisle two by two like animals boarding Noah's ark. I am fully and deeply engaged in a wholly different way. Despite the traditional song of marriage sung in chorus by my well-wishing southern aunts, I have different ambitions. I am otherwise engaged.

> *Here we can see that the student is going to go with*
> *a theme of "engaged" for this personal statement.*
> *As a reader, I'm already frustrated by it.*

I learned at a young age to be fully engaged in every activity and be present in everything I did. My interests have always been teasingly diverse. My areas of study in college proved the same. My passions continued to pull me in unconventional directions. Many friends, family members and career counselors advised me to choose a singular course of study. However, multitasking had always been a significant part of my life and I wanted to take advantage of the opportunity to pursue my multifaceted passions. Having a major in biology with a premed emphasis and a minor in dance afforded me the chance to challenge my mind and body. As a member of the dance company, I often found myself racing between a ballet class and labs like comparative anatomy where I had to quickly change my focus to performing a precise dissection, even if it was in a leotard. The physical and academic challenges these two distinct disciplines presented have prepared me for the rigorous requirements of being a physician. I know as I move forward and play the many roles a doctor must play my ability to engage fully in each task will set me apart.

> *The student introduces us to the fact that she majored in biology, and she was a premed student. Why? I want to know why not just what. She also compares her rigorous journey to that of being a physician, which doesn't belong in a personal statement. How does she know about the "many roles a doctor must play?" This paragraph doesn't add anything.*

People are another passion of mine. Whether it is giving a tour of my school, talking with new moms at the women's clinic or answering questions at research symposiums; engaging with others has always fueled me. In my lifetime I want to connect with people around me and affect my community in a positive way. I was given such an opportunity when I heard about a medical mission study abroad trip to El Salvador through my University. Participants would be given the chance to work in hospitals and learn what medicine looked like in an undeveloped country with rudimentary medical resources. At the time only nursing students were invited. However, I used my persuasive skills to gain the first premed spot on the trip organizing opportunities to shadow medical professionals and observe surgeries. My enthusiasm faded when I saw how much direct contact the nursing students had with patients and wondered if I had possibly chosen the wrong career path. I also saw how warm and open they were with their emotions. I deeply admired them for their contribution but feared I wasn't demonstrative enough for a healthcare career. Clarity came as I witnessed a doctor frantically looked for women to join him in an examination room to do a breast exam on a patient who had obvious lumps protruding from her chest. The other nurses became emotional at the very difficult sight but I was able to rise to the occasion and approached the situation in an emotionally different way. I realized at that moment my niche to serve and that I had the strength to engage differently and effectively. I discovered that what I thought was my weakness was my strength.

The student writes a lot about a clinical experience in this paragraph. She tries to sneak in a pitch about her "persuasive" skills, but I'm not sure what that has to do with being a physician. I got a little lost when the student wrote about not being demonstrative enough and she wondered if she had chosen the wrong career path. I'm not sure what skills or traits she thinks she needs to have to be a physician. I could read this and think that the student lacks empathy because she did not empathize with the patient or have any feelings about her situation, in contrast to the nursing students who were also there.

I was also able to extend my service to countries like El Salvador through my research at State University where I worked on better understanding a vector of malaria's circulatory and immune system. I committed many grueling hours using a tiny needle to inject mosquitoes with a dose of neuropeptide. Two accidental releases of mosquitoes, 6 bites later and what seemed like a hundred imperfect sticks to their abdomen, I was ready to be done with the whole project. But the work was so important to me that I remained engaged in the bigger picture, stayed persistent, and wore long sleeve shirts. My commitment paid off, as I became a published author in The Journal of Experimental Biology. While this experience taught me a lot about the scientific process and how to investigate problems from different angles I knew my greatest passion was still working with my own species.

Having experience with research is a good thing. It's not required as a premed, but it's good to have exposure to it. I personally don't think research should be written about in a personal statement unless there is something unique or some prestigious award that you received from it. Research is a part of being a physician, and you'll probably do some form of research during medical school or residency. To me, doing research doesn't add enough to your story about why you want to be a physician to include it.

Persistence and "grit" became a common theme in my quest to become a doctor. So much so that I began to acclimate to the bumpy ride and just buckle up. The largest hurdle I experienced was my first attempt at the MCAT. After receiving my first score I was faced with the possibility that my greatest dream may not become a reality. An advisor told me that I was at the end of my road. The thought of losing my dream felt like losing a limb. I knew that becoming a doctor is more than a dream to me, it is part of who I am. I rejected the notion that I was at the end of my road in pursuing my passion of becoming a doctor. I was determined to fully engage myself to retake the MCAT and achieve my dreams.

This is a red flag statement. As I mentioned in the red flag chapter, not doing well on the MCAT is not a big enough red flag to mention in your personal statement.

I don't have a precious gem on my finger. But I am engaged. I have declared an oath to my passion, to fulfill my deep desire to engage with patients as a physician. Despite the many obstacles I have faced and those yet to come, I know that I will remain focused on achieving my goal so that I can further positively affect the world around me. Someday I hope to get engaged in the traditional sense but for now I am otherwise engaged.

The student brings it back to the "engaged" theme that she has continued throughout the personal statement. I counted engaged, in different forms, sixteen times throughout the essay.
She makes a statement here as well about the "many obstacles" she encountered. She only mentioned the MCAT in her personal statement, so I'm left wondering what else there may be.
This is a great example of a student trying too hard to theme a personal statement and missing the mark about showing me why she wants to be a physician. You can read her final draft next.

TJ FINAL DRAFT

My retinas burned as they filled with flashing red and white lights piercing through the cloud of gravel dust engulfing us. Sitting in my driveway was an ambulance and my mother was inside. I could feel the ground that had always felt so steady under my feet begin to tremble. The weeks following, I struggled to grasp medical jargon, and tried to suppress my alarm as foreboding wires weaved like eerie vines entrapping my mother. In a sea of confusion I was comforted by the one thing I could understand as a 9-year-old; our family physician's persistent dedication to our family. I remember standing in the hospital room feeling useless. As a problem solver I wanted nothing more than to fix my mom, but I couldn't. From that day forward I wanted to do whatever was necessary to gain the tools to be able to heal others like I wasn't able to do for my mother. My frustration led to motivation. When the dust settled, I began to sense that I had gained an inner strength from a seed of passion that had been planted during the chaos.

This is a great opening paragraph that illustrates an atmosphere of chaos in a young 9-year-old's life. It's an excellent showing paragraph. We're immediately given the "seed." In fact, the student even called it a seed.

From the rubble that lingered, my life began to take shape. I wanted to be the person that in a time of such instability in a family's foundation would be an anchor; working diligently to find what truly lay beneath the surface. This newfound purpose was now guiding decisions in my life from as small as having my mother make a white coat out of one of my dad's old dress shirts for career day to spending my summers as a volunteer with the University Hospital's Teen Summer Volunteer Program.

> *The student writes about the newfound purpose she mentioned in the previous paragraph, which leads to one of her first memorable volunteering experiences.*

One day while volunteering, a nurse said she desperately needed help in one of the rooms. I followed her down the hall; her words trailing behind her. "She is a young mom with no family helping her, with a very sick baby who is fussy. We need you to hold the baby while she goes out for a smoke break." I paused, looking at the baby screaming in her crib, I hadn't had a lot of experience with infants and was a little apprehensive. I was immediately reminded of my mother as I saw the little baby veiled in wires and tubes. I reached down and cradled the delicate baby in my arms. I could feel my nervousness making my movements rigid as I carefully tried to avoid disrupting the babies' many attachments. I began to sing, both to comfort the baby and myself. As time passed and I relaxed, so did the baby. We soon swayed in silence as her eyelids grew heavy and began to close. I had felt what it was like to, in the smallest way, comfort a family member when chaos consumed them. This experience ignited my desire to do this not only in the summers as a volunteer but every day as a physician.

> *"I paused, looking at the baby screaming in her crib." This is a* showing *statement. The student could have easily written "the baby was screaming in her crib," but it would haven't have been as good of a sentence. The student paints a picture of wires and tubes and describes the memory of her mother in a similar situation.*

A few years later I again found myself in a hospital, this time in El Salvador on a study abroad trip. I felt the room fill with the hot, wet air. A frantic doctor surged through the door ushering in a woman slightly hunched over. She shuffled along with her eyes glued to the floor. Under her top were obvious lumps coming from an abnormally shaped female chest. My heart broke as even someone without much medical experience could see she had visible tumors all over her concave chest. In broken English the doctor begged for someone to be present for a breast examination as El Salvador culture had very strict regulations about men being alone with members of the opposite sex.

> *Again, this is an excellent* showing *paragraph. Writing "A frantic doctor surged through the door ushering in a woman slightly hunched over" forces me to* see *what is going on. If she had written "the doctor came into the room with a woman," it wouldn't have been as memorable.*

The doctor, the woman and I entered the primitive exam room. She sat on a bench as he began explaining the examination. The woman's hunched back made it difficult for her to look up so her eyes never met his. The woman's fear was palpable. I could see her began to pull away from the doctors outreached hand. I squatted down beside her to get on eye level with her. For the first time her brown eyes met mine. I watched as the fear in her body began to soften. The doctor's hand moved across her chest and I watched as it moved over each protrusion. I may not have been able to speak her language, but I knew what it felt like to be vulnerable. I kept my eyes on hers and softly smiled as I attempted to comfort her. This experience humbled me and gave me even more motivation to continue working towards the goal of becoming a physician. Someday, I hope to experience the honor of patients giving me their trust and using it to comfort them and hopefully bring healing.

> *The student continues to evoke the room, the physician, and the patient. She* shows, *through the use of her words, that she is compassionate. She doesn't need to* tell *me that she is compassionate; she just* showed *me by describing keeping her eyes on the patient and smiling softly. She finishes with a great takeaway about how this experience has motivated her to continue down this path.*

Chaos is often something we fear. Instability can cause things to fall. In my case, the instability I have experienced in my life due to my mother's health made way for a purpose to fall into place. I was shaped by my mother's illness, sculpted by holding that sweet infant and transformed by the fragile El Salvadorian woman. The trust patients have so carefully given to me in my limited medical experience has molded my motivation to pursue my goal of becoming a physician no matter the obstacle. I hope to gain further knowledge and skills to earn the privilege of my patient's trust and humbly act as their guardian and advocate in their most vulnerable, shaken state.

The student does a great job of bringing everything together in this final paragraph. She has added some creative flourishes, but she didn't go overboard with them. She outlines what she hopes to accomplish as a physician.

This student was able to do a complete 180 from her first draft. It only took a couple of drafts after the first one to get to this point.

"Best personal statement ever." This was the feedback from the Dean of Admissions at a Midwestern allopathic school. He interviewed this student and told her it was the best he had ever read.

Not surprisingly, she was accepted.

JW FINAL DRAFT

I stood up from my desk and tried again, repeating the lines that were burned into my brain from hours of repetition and rehearsal. I imagined the hunger pangs that pierced my abdomen, the dull headache, the weakness in my limbs, and the utter exhaustion of my spirit. I was long past the memorization stage and now onto discovering how to make the playwright's words come alive. I had to discover how to infuse my performance with the physicality brought about by chronic starvation and the mental anguish from being imprisoned without an end in sight. I was fortunate enough to have the lead role, Fania Fenelon, in the production of Playing for Time by Arthur Miller. The play was based on the true story of Fania, a French singer using her musical talent to survive Auschwitz during WWII. It was my job to bring her truth to my performance and honor her story.

> *This opening draws me in, causing me to wonder who the student is and what she is going to tell me. It does a great job of* showing *and not* telling. *After reading this, I'm assuming this student is a nontraditional premed.*

This was my favorite part of the rehearsal process. As a child and young adult, I loved school. In the acting world, this translated into a love of researching a role and doing script analysis. A genuine curiosity about the human psyche is what drew me to the acting profession. On stages in New York City and Los Angeles, I had the opportunity to explore characters written by playwrights such as Bertolt Brecht, William Shakespeare, and Patrick Marber. Not only were these experiences artistically satisfying, they taught me valuable skills such as remaining calm under pressure, overcoming anxiety, and being comfortable in front of people.

> *She has now confirmed that she is a nontraditional student, and previously she was an actress. Immediately I am interested because she is unique. This is one of the benefits of being a nontraditional premed student.*

Despite the wonderful experiences I had while acting, I did not feel fulfilled. I realized that I longed for a career in which I could have a direct impact on people's lives. After watching Dr. H fight for my father's quality of life, I began to realize that a career in medicine might be a perfect fit for me. My father's stage III colon cancer diagnosis was unexpected and devastating. When the surgeon suggested removing his entire colon for preventive reasons, Dr. H, my father's gastroenterologist, fought against it. This type of surgery would result in the need for a colostomy bag, something my father wanted to avoid if possible. The surgeon eventually yielded to Dr. H, removing only the cancerous region of his colon. Years later, my father's cancer is still in remission and he is back to living an active lifestyle. This experience taught me the humbling nature of disease and the stress it places on patients and their families. Furthermore, I learned the importance of patient advocacy. Dr. H fought for my father's dignity when the rest of my family was too blinded by fear to even consider an alternative. I knew then that I wanted to be able to help people in ways that only a physician can. I knew that this is the kind of physician I wanted to become. I sought out clinical experiences to gain a deeper understanding of the medical field and to ensure that this was truly a path I wanted to pursue. These clinical experiences solidified my desire to become a physician.

> *"I knew then that I wanted to be able to help people in ways that only a physician can." This is a very direct, and very powerful takeaway. The student is showing me, without hesitation, "I need to be a physician." The student highlights the "seed" that was planted for her and why it affected her.*

"You should go talk to M. She was an actress, just like you!" Per the charge nurse's instructions, I knocked on M's door. I introduced myself as a volunteer and asked if she would be willing to participate in a patient feedback survey. She paused and then burst into tears. I stood in the doorway and said, "I'm not just here for the survey. I can also listen if you need someone to talk to." M told me that none of her friends had come to visit, she just found out she had cancer, and an hour ago she received an IRS notice which would bankrupt her. Her world was crumbling around her and she did not see a point in continuing on. I did not say much; I held her hand and listened. A few months prior, I had shadowed Dr. N in Palliative Care. He stressed the importance of attending to a patient's emotional pain in addition to their physical pain. I was not qualified to help M with her physical pain; however, I was able to attend to her emotional pain. I spent over two hours in the room with M. When I left the room, she seemed more at ease. I informed her nurse of our conversation. We discussed the holistic approach to patient care, which requires addressing the patient's mental anguish in addition to their physical discomfort. I learned the importance of inquiring about a patient's life and background in addition to the physical symptoms they present with. I walked away from my shift that night knowing in my heart that I made the right decision to change careers. A career in medicine offers a lifetime of rewarding work, allowing you to be there for people during their times of greatest need.

This student effectively illuminates an interaction with a patient, the impact that she had on that patient, as well as the impact the patient had on her. She has a great takeaway that, "I made the right decision to change careers." The last sentence could have probably been removed since it's telling me what a career in medicine is like.

I spent years pursuing the artistic exploration of the human psyche; now I am switching my focus to the scientific exploration of the human brain and body. My career as an actress has equipped me with valuable skills that I can use as a physician. Furthermore, my personal and clinical experiences have inspired me to become a compassionate physician who considers both the benefits and consequences of medical treatment. I have played many roles in my acting career; however, a career as a physician will allow me to simultaneously take on all the roles I desire: a researcher, a lifelong learner, a mentor, an advocate, and a healer.

This is a strong conclusion, with the student writing about focusing on the "scientific exploration of the human brain and body."
She could have expanded this to explain how she wants to impact future patients. There are some good tie-ins with acting and artistry that she makes as well that don't feel forced. This is a great personal statement that really makes me want to invite her for an interview. This student was invited to many interviews, and she is attending an allopathic medical school in the Mid-Atlantic region.

DM FINAL DRAFT

My journey to medical school began with an existential crisis after my 2005 deployment to Afghanistan. When my unit arrived, we were in what was known as the most dangerous place in Afghanistan. The constant threat to my life, and the deaths of seven comrades from my company, made me face the possibility that I might not make it back alive. At the last stop before home, I stopped to stare at the January sky. I wanted to remember that moment because I finally felt safe. When I finally got home, the euphoria of being alive was replaced by survivor's guilt. I learned that one way I could resolve my feelings of guilt and honor my fallen brothers was to make the most of my life.

> *This student hits you hard with a nontraditional story*
> *of being a soldier. It makes me want to keep reading.*

In 2007, I deployed again to Afghanistan. I translated between the medical staff in our mobile clinic and Iraqi mothers with children suffering from spina bifida. The mothers were desperate and begging for help. Spina bifida was a death sentence in Afghanistan since the country lacked the specialized medical facilities to treat these children. The staff was only able to give each child a health assessment and referrals for treatment outside of Afghanistan. Despite the meager treatment options available, the mothers entered the clinic with despair and left grateful and full of hope. I trained as an infantryman to cause bodily harm to the enemy, yet here I was taking part in a process meant to heal and rehabilitate people. The experience was profoundly gratifying because I witnessed a moment of joy in a city full of despair.

> *The student describes being a translator at a clinic, interacting with physicians, patients, and their mothers. It's a great story highlighting his initial "seed."*

Being at the clinic was the first time I considered working in healthcare. However, I did not think it would be an obtainable goal because I struggled academically in high school due to undiagnosed Attention Deficit Hyperactive Disorder (ADHD). In the Army, I was treated for ADHD and gained the discipline and maturity I lacked in high school. After the Army, I started college with no set goals or expectations, yet as I progressed with my degree in psychology, I became more confident in my academic abilities. My discipline and maturity turned education from a chore to a passion for knowledge.

> *The student offers information about a mental health disorder. This is always a slippery slope for a personal statement. You risk me saying, "it's not worth the gamble" and putting your application aside. That said, I think this paragraph excels in explaining why the student went into the Army first, and how he has a newfound love for learning.*

In my senior year, I started a research work-study with the Department of Veteran Affairs (VA). I contributed to two research studies: enrollment of rural veterans into VA healthcare and a comparative analysis of the quality of primary care for the homeless. I gained a better understanding of the demands and unique healthcare needs of both rural veterans and the homeless population. I felt satisfaction in knowing that I played a role in conducting research that would one day help address the healthcare needs of my fellow veterans. After graduating, I worked for seven months as a mental health technician for the VA in Tennessee. I valued the opportunity to work with fellow veterans and the experience I gained from working on a clinical team, but I felt limited due to my non-clinical support role. I wanted to have a more active role in healthcare and decided to set my goal on becoming a physician. The journey would be long and challenging, but I knew that the discipline and drive I developed in the Army would allow me to succeed.

This paragraph leads to the kind of "wanting more" type statement we've talked about before. It would have been stronger if he had told me a story of working with one of the patients and how he wanted to help that patient more.

With new purpose, I moved back to Alabama to commit to entering medical school. In the summer of 2014, I shadowed at the Acute Care for Elderly at the University of Alabama at Birmingham hospital. The unique demands of geriatric care, coupled with the work of the interdisciplinary care team, piqued my interest in this field of medicine. I then volunteered at the Birmingham VA Medical Center by transporting patients to surgery. The experiences I had there were especially rewarding, as I had the privilege to meet other veterans and hear their unique stories.

This paragraph highlights two different extracurricular activities and probably could have been cut to save room for a good story about a patient.

My journey from Infantryman to a hopeful doctor has come full circle. In the past, my duties were to protect this country by causing harm, and now I find myself on a path where I will do no harm. I began not knowing where or who I would be in the future. I now know that I must keep my promise to give purpose to my life as a way of honoring my fallen friends and continuing to serve my community, be it veterans or the rural community in which I live.

This is a really good conclusion. The student has a great line about going from causing harm in the Army to doing no harm as a physician. He has a clear mission of honoring his fallen friends and serving the community. Overall, this personal statement is effective in showing me why. It also gives me some information about his nontraditional past, which helps him stand out.
This student is attending an allopathic medical school in the South.

DB FINAL DRAFT

Sprinting from a beating helicopter and fighting to see through the dust and night vision goggles in the middle of the night in Southern Iraq, I was doing everything I could to clear a safe path for my strike force. Trying to see through the grit was like trying to blink away sweat while opening the door to a hot oven. I had to push the pace; speed and surprise were our best security in raids like these. I didn't feel like a "barrel-chested freedom fighter"; I initially felt like an impostor. I was an Army special operations explosive ordnance disposal team leader, and I was absolutely terrified. What was I doing here? How did I find myself in this position, responsible for this many lives? I was as scared as I have ever been. Along with 60 strangers that I had met only hours before, we made it through the region of the world most densely laden with improvised explosive devices that night; it was the first of many.

> *I used this example previously in the book.*
> *It's a great* showing *paragraph that gets you using your senses.*
> *You feel like you're the one running from the helicopter.*

An incredible amount of anticipation led up to that moment. A similar sense of angst started building a couple years into that assignment. I was set to separate from active duty in a mere 20 months, after what would be nearly 8 years of service. I hungered for more intellectual stimulation. The cyclic nature of deployment, training events, and returns to Iraq proved to be unsustainable for both me and my wife. However, I was almost equally as torn with the prospect of completing a business degree and searching for a job. What was I going to do with "just a job?" I needed the next challenge - one that would provide similar instances to serve, a strong sense of teamwork, and continue to deliver learning opportunities.

The student drives home the fact that he's a nontraditional student with eight years of service in the Army and explains that he is looking for the next "challenge." At first, reading this, I'm a little concerned— it's like medicine is just something to conquer. So I'll keep reading and see what is really motivating him.

I distinctly remember the conversation with my wife while we were on vacation. I was less than a week removed from Iraq, and my final deployment loomed on the calendar ahead. I finally mustered the courage the be blunt with her and explain my predicament. I tried to put myself in her position, having caught this curveball that I had just thrown her way. She replied to my utter surprise, "Finally!" Along with a brief motivational speech and supportive endorsement to pursue whatever I wish followed, so long as I do so with the same intensity that made me the person I was in the military. A once fleeting thought I had some time before that conversation was suddenly given the spark it needed.

This paragraph doesn't tell me much other than that the student had a conversation with his wife. It could have been left out if information was needed to flesh out other stories.

I had known my wife's best friend Amy for some time, first meeting her during her final year of medical school when she was in her early 30's. Her excitement in finding something she loved and challenged her after changing careers was always palpable. Now, 4 years later, I found myself seriously considering something I had once written off as impossible. I had previously considered medicine years ago, but this was the first time I did so with maturity, drive and a sense of self. Having completed residency, Amy gave me the most complete picture possible of what being a physician means, as well as the steps required to get there. After our discussions, my own research, and months of deliberation, I felt strongly that I had made the right choice. This was the only path I could be absolutely passionate about, would deliver the challenges I was looking for, and provide opportunities to continue serving others in their time of need.

"I had previously considered medicine years ago." We've talked about these types of statements before. This leaves me asking "when?" and "why?" What led you to consider medicine years ago? The student rushed from the decision to choose medicine into "discussions," "research," and "months of deliberation." He knew it was the "only path." The core of the personal statement is discussing this journey, and he squished it down into two sentences.

The biggest obstacle I faced would be to repair whatever damage I could to my running academic record. My initial foray into higher education ten years ago was devoid of any sense of responsibility. Deciding to pursue medical school marked a turning point in both focus and drive in academics. I knew demonstrating the potential to succeed academically in medical school is a prerequisite. I was fortunate to be allowed to enroll in 16 hours of basic sciences during the final months of my service obligation while conducting night training for new trainees. That initial science coursework was my final self-test to prove my dream could be feasible. I knew shortly after beginning those courses that I would be alright. I have since completed 67 credit hours with a 3.95 GPA, 58 of those hours in science and math. I was always superficially interested with science and technology, but I have become enthralled with learning since focusing on a degree in biochemistry.

The student brings up a red flag, but then writes a lot about the hours of credit he completed and the GPA he accomplished. This is in the application and doesn't need to be in the personal statement.

Now, one year separated from active duty and over two years after committing myself to this path, I am more confident than ever that I have made the right decision. Physician shadowing and clinical experiences solidified the foundation I was building. My time in the military gave me a unique perspective, but the things I loved about my job came at a brutal price. Although well worth the personal sacrifice, the thrill of the unknown and the sense of service to my partners took place in an unsustainable setting. I believe and hope that medicine will provide a similar sense of camaraderie, appreciation for life, and humbling opportunities to serve others, while also knowing that those occasions will ultimately be for the right reasons; that the personal sacrifices will unequivocally be for the greater good. I know medical school is only the beginning of a very long and difficult path, but, in my experience, the difficult path has always been worth the sacrifice.

Here, the student writes about shadowing a physician and clinical experience. I'd love to hear why those experiences "solidified the foundation." This is telling, not showing. What is the next step? What is the goal once he becomes a physician? Ultimately, this is an okay personal statement. It's missing the all-important why. The student told me he went on a journey of discovery but didn't tell us about it.
That said, I think the student really stands out because of his background, and that alone would have intrigued me enough to want to interview him.
This student is attending an allopathic medical school in the South.

KL FINAL DRAFT

"John? John?!" I heard the receptionist yell desperately from the front of the cosmetics manufacturing company where I am a senior manufacturing engineer. I bolted out into the hallway to find John, one of the salespeople, lying motionless face down in the hallway. I sprinted down the hallway and knelt by his side. He did not appear to be breathing. Preparing for the worst, I rolled him over while the people around me frantically worked to call 911. Relief flooded through me as John began taking in great gasps of air. He also began to convulse. Drawing on prior knowledge from a number of sources, I rolled him over on his side, held him firmly until his seizure subsided, talked to him clearly and calmly as he came to and attempted to keep him lying down. When he unsteadily struggled to his feet despite my persuasions, I held him firmly from behind speaking to him calmly and compassionately while pinning his arms down until the paramedics arrived. Afterward the owner thanked me profusely. When I stated, "I only did what anyone else would do," she looked at me and said sincerely, "No, most people would not have done that."

> *I'm greeted right at the start with an interesting story of an encounter the student had. We're not sure what to make of it yet though because there isn't a takeaway. It may be stronger with a takeaway, but it serves its purpose by making me want to keep reading.*

It never crossed my mind that someone could come out into that hallway and see someone else lying helpless, perhaps dying, on the floor and not immediately take action. Her words had two profound effects on me. First, they made me reflect on why I was compelled to act at the site of a fellow human being in need. I possessed innate tendencies to help my fellow man. This also explained why I felt such a strong pull to leave my successful career and pursue the path of a physician. Though I had made the decision a year earlier, this realization further concreted my choice. Medicine was where I belonged; I was working toward becoming what I was meant to be.

> *Here we get the takeaway. It's a longer one, and a potent one, so it's okay that it's not at the end of the previous paragraph. In this paragraph, we learn that the student is a nontraditional student. He used a powerful word that I've written about a lot in this book—reflection. He reflected on his experience. This is a very nice piece to add to a personal statement. It doesn't have to be that exact word, but the act of reflecting in some way can take a good personal statement to greatness.*

Secondly, her words reminded me just how far I had come from that dark, cold road in Brooklyn 12 years prior in January of 2003. I was team leader of a road crew for my company. We had been traveling for months working onsite at post offices from 6:00 pm to 6:00 am upgrading thousands of postal vehicles. My team was proud to be recognized as first in productivity of the 16 teams just like it blanketing the U.S. En route to our 3rd Brooklyn post office of the night we came across a body lying in the road. We pulled over and slowly approached it, stopping about 10 feet short. Steam was slowly rising from the man but no breath could be seen. I was petrified. My feet refused to move and I stayed rooted in place until the police arrived. It was a hit and run. The man was pronounced dead. Ever since, though there was probably nothing I could have done, that moment has haunted me. That man may have laid there and died while I stood at a distance and watched.

> *This paragraph illustrates a different encounter with a situation from the student's past. This time he didn't act. Again, we're not given a takeaway, so I'm not sure what to make of the story.*

That same road crew took me from Detroit to New Jersey to Florida and all the way to California. My heart ached for the victims at ground zero, I was shocked by the slums of Detroit, I stood amazed by the ocean in Florida and I felt exhilaration free falling 14,000 feet above California. I attended a new church every week: Methodist, Protestant, Vineyard, Catholic and Southern Baptist to name a few (the last being the most memorable). These experiences left me with a deeper sense of community and diversity. Still, my most poignant experience was on assignment in Mexico.

> *The student highlights some of his experiences as a nontraditional student, but I've yet to see a true* why medicine *statement.*

As a manufacturing engineer, I was tasked with launching a factory to build vehicles for a large corporate contract. Nothing could have prepared me for what was to come. Upon arrival the challenge became clear. No one there spoke English, and my coworker and I spoke very little Spanish. The "factory" was a dirt lot in the slums of Mexico surrounded by concrete walls and barbed wire with a haphazard tin roof. Families lived in the lot and dogs and children ran around while workers welded, sawed and riveted. We had to unload semi-trucks with 12 men, a rope and a front-end loader. Still, they were happy. We exceeded our productivity goals by 30% and those men gave me a present that will last a lifetime; the awareness that to be alive is a gift and each day is an opportunity.

> *I'm given more details about the student's nontraditional past. This could easily be an extracurricular description.*

I have not always taken advantage of those opportunities given to me. However, I do believe that the course of my life has prepared me to make the most of them now. Starting with my keen interest in technology at a very young age I have always had a longstanding desire to be at the cutting edge of advancement. That drive, coupled with my rich professional experience and a yearning to help people in need, has made my path clear to me. To become a physician will fulfill these desires. It would be a great honor to be granted the opportunity to enter this path and one which I do not think any single individual is completely worthy of or prepared for. There is no greater calling than to spend each day making a difference to people through treatment, understanding and caring. I have had the amazing opportunity to shadow two physicians, Dr. Smith and Dr. Johnson, who have exemplified this attitude in daily practice. Through them I have seen what it is to approach patients with respect, sympathy and kindness. That is the kind of physician I want to be. The kind of man I want to be. Never again will I look back and say I stopped ten feet short.

This last paragraph finally gives us a hint that the student wants to be a physician and shares with us some of the experiences that have strengthened that vision. He writes about his nontraditional past and how he hopes his interests will meld in the future as a physician. He writes about shadowing and the impact the physicians had on him.

What makes this student stand out is all of the stories he told as a nontraditional student. This personal statement doesn't follow the advice I've given in this book, but I wanted to include it to show the diversity of statements that work. What makes this personal statement stand out is how personal *it is. It could be much more powerful if he included a little bit more about a patient experience. I still don't know if he likes being around patients. I have to assume that and read his extracurricular descriptions to learn more. The student also probably did well on his secondary essays to get interviews at medical schools and ultimately an acceptance at a great allopathic school in the South.*

One other note about this student and essay. This student had a huge red flag in his application; he was academically dismissed. He didn't write about it here, but he did mention it in his secondaries. Specifically, he wrote, "I opted to not discuss my academic dismissal in my personal statement as I felt that the few words I was allowed would be better spent painting a picture of who I am and I let my grade record do the talking."

JR FINAL DRAFT

My grandfather once told me that time is the greatest healer. I learned what he meant by that in the summer of 2010. My phone rang at lunch and I was notified that my grandfather was in a horrific oil well explosion. I made it to the hospital in time to say goodbye, but I was still in shock over the events of the last several months. September 2009 had marked the legal end of my marriage and that of my parents; neither of which were expected. My once foundational safety net suddenly disintegrated.

The student leads us into his story through a tragedy. The last sentence is powerful and makes me want to see what happens next.

Following the culmination of these events I found myself working in the Oklahoma oilfields as I needed to step back from everything to reset my life. Later in the summer of 2010 I was making a run to New York to pick up a boat for some extra money. By nightfall I was in Indianapolis looking for the nearest hotel. I found myself walking into a hotel partnered with a major hospital and medical school. I checked into my room and attempted to get some sleep. I felt restless. I looked out my window and watched the hustle and bustle of the hospital. After observing the doctors, medical students, and nurses hurriedly entering and exiting the hospital's large revolving glass doors, my heart started to beat out of my chest. Call it an epiphany but right at that moment I knew I had come full circle. I had an overwhelming sense of illumination in my heart and soul. That moment I began formulating a game plan to achieve my passion and my calling which had never left my heart: that of being a physician.

Plan in place I returned to college spring 2012 and shortly after started working fulltime as a phlebotomist at Norman Regional Hospital while going to school. One particular day stands out above all others. My shift started at three a.m.; the units were overly packed with lab orders, and we were shorthanded. I had to draw blood on about thirty patients before six a.m. Anything that seemed possible that day to go wrong seemed to go completely wrong. Patients were disgruntled at the four a.m. needle stick wake up call, nurses were barking additional lab orders, physicians were frustrated that labs weren't drawn earlier, and so on.

We've seen several students now make the same mistake of referring to a previous passion for becoming a physician without properly expanding on it. Here the student describes witnessing the "hustle and bustle" of the hospital and formulating a plan to "achieve my passion and my calling which had never left my heart." Where did that come from? Why was that there? This will always be the question I ask if you vaguely state that this is your passion without providing a reason for that passion. You can't water the seed without first planting it.

The morning continued dragging on and there just seemed to be no end in sight. Later during my lunch break I had received orders to draw blood on an elderly female patient, "we'll call her Mrs. Smith". I was very frustrated at that point because I hadn't had time for a drink of water or a snack for energy. I needed a moment to regroup from the fragmented morning.

The student conveys the chaotic morning well. It could have been shortened, however, to get to the good stuff, which is the actual patient interaction with Mrs. Smith. You don't need to put statements like "we'll call her Mrs. Smith" in your personal statement. Just use generic first names, and you'll be fine.

I left my hunger in the cafeteria, took the order and proceeded to the patient's room. Though I felt no angst toward my patient, it would be understandable if Mrs. Smith saw me as a tired and grumpy phlebotomist. As I was drawing her blood, Mrs. Smith used her free arm and put something into my top scrub breast pocket. I finished drawing her blood and looked to see what she had put in my pocket. It was a candycane decorated to resemble a reindeer. She then told me how much she appreciated the good job I had done by having the needle stick hardly hurt and that she was very thankful for me.

> *Here we see the impact a patient had on the student and the impact the student had on the patient. What is missing is the takeaway. Why did this experience further his desire to be a physician?*

To say the least I was very shocked. All I did was draw her blood. I wasn't the one helping her get better or curing her ailment. For this patient to be so thankful for me to just draw her blood really hit me pretty hard in how ungrateful an attitude I had all that day. I wished her the best and thanked her for the reindeer candycane.

> *I don't know what this is adding to the personal statement. It probably could be cut without hurting the overall story. Cutting a paragraph or sentence is a very good test to see if it changes the story or your personal statement. Delete it, save it as a new copy (don't forget to save the old copy) and have someone read it to see if it still makes sense.*

Pondering upon the experience further, I realized that this is what I love about medicine and why I want to be a physician. It is the human interaction, experience of healing others, and making a direct tangible impact upon those seeking help. When I feel stressed, demoralized, or beaten down on this long road to becoming a physician I look at the reindeer candycane that I keep on my desk and remember this experience. It serves to remind me of why I am doing this.

This is a great takeaway paragraph explaining why medicine. It specifically identifies "human interaction," "healing others," and "making a direct tangible impact" on patients.

As an eight-year-old following my father on medical rounds through his clinic I knew deeply then that I wanted to be a physician. I started on a linear path and then the curvature of circumstances and consequences occurred. It has been these artifacts on my lifeline that now show up as my greatest pinnacles of success. It is my belief that, allowed to direct the totality of my personal energy to the study of medicine my ability to succeed cannot be doubted.

Okay, so his father was a physician. This would have been great information to have earlier. When he wrote about always having the passion, I asked, "Where did that come from?"
Now we know. The student tries to get a little fancy with his words, writing about a "linear path" and a "curvature of circumstances." Fancy words and descriptions are often not needed. Use simple words. Easy to understand sentences help me understand, in a concise way, what you are trying to accomplish.
At the end of this personal statement, I'm able to put it all together and get a good picture of who this student is. It took me a little work to put it together, but it's all there. With a few small tweaks, this would have been a great personal statement. As it is, it was good enough to get the student several interviews.
This student is attending an osteopathic medical school in the Midwest.

LR EARLY DRAFT

Growing up, I was always considered the dreamer of the family. I saw everything through the famed rose-colored glasses and did not believe in limits. My career goals included everything from President to entertainer to physician. But as I got older, I realized I didn't want to center my life around politics and that I had no desire to overcome stage fright. However, my interest in the well-being of others and love for scientific knowledge only increased. So I set my eyes on the goal – study Biology, get that degree and jump right into medical school. Little did I know how those rose-colored glasses would be damaged along the way. It seemed as if every time the lenses would grow foggy in the face of adversity, I would attempt to clean them, only to return them to my face and find them scratched and cracked just a little more, until I could no longer see out of them.

Similar to the previous student, we're given a mission statement type opening. Of note here is that the student based her discussion around the theme of rose-colored glasses. In my mind, I'm bracing myself to read a personal statement based on this theme. That's not a good thing. We're given her reason for wanting to be a doctor—a love for scientific knowledge. This is not a reason to be a physician. To satisfy a love for science, you can be a science teacher, a PhD researcher, an engineer, or any number of other careers.

From freshman year to the Spring of my fourth year, depression consumed me. Slowly, I began forging my own limits for myself and attached them to me like a prisoner's chain. At the peak of this season, and easily the lowest time in my life, my long-term relationship had turned emotionally abusive and I was put out of my home because of said relationship. I was sleeping 14+ hours a day in a house that I couldn't call home and barely getting by in class. I had convinced myself I would never be good enough for medical school. After failing my third Chemistry test for the semester, I decided to go seek help from my professor. Though the conversation had no impact on my grade, it was the best decision I'd made since I started college. I was directed to a case manager and therapist at the school who taught me that it was okay! I was okay, depression was okay and that my career would be okay! Don't get me wrong, my life did not change instantaneously. I still had to find my own place, learn study skills and recover information I'd studied but not learned. But I was able to see a goal and remove some of those links from the chain around my waist.

There are some interesting points in this paragraph. The first one is the student discussing a potential red flag—her depression. She is using it to explain her poor grades and discuss what was going on in her life. I think this is okay. Mental health disorders can be tricky to navigate, and you certainly don't want to give a reader any reason to reject you, but I think the student did this appropriately here.

The second interesting aspect that I would tell you to avoid is the language she used in speaking directly to me. She said, "don't get me wrong." This type of writing is awkward in a personal statement and should be avoided.

So now was the time to reconsider medicine. Volunteering, shadowing and research all began but I found myself still asking the most essential question – why medicine? I could never find the right answer until one day when I was sitting down to breakfast in my mother's new home after making pancakes with a homemade blackberry syrup to go on top. The meal was so picture-perfect that I pulled up Facebook, thinking I would share it with everyone. As I was thumbing through the newsfeed I saw him – Onmar, a five-year-old boy whose family home fell victim to a bomb in war-torn Syria. The video shows little Onmar being put into an ambulance, in complete shock, coated in concrete dust with blood pouring from his hairline, which he doesn't even notice until he wipes his eyes. He stared blankly out from his seat, probably trying to figure out what happened with what little vocabulary he has learned in his 5 short years. In that moment my soul longed to get on a plane, armed with only the compassion in my heart and the knowledge of medicine to heal their wounds and let them know that not all of this world and someone wants to take care of them. In this moment, part of my life was changed instantaneously. My thoughts were thrown back to that child I left behind so many years ago who refused to accept a limitation and believed it was impossible to truly try and fail. I knew that to whom much is given, much is expected, and lived by the quote, "your talent is God's gift to you. What you do with it is your gift back to God" by Leo Buscaglia. So I picked up a brand new pair of rose-colored glasses and set out to finish what I started so many years ago. Yes, I have absolutely made mistakes along the way. Yes, there have absolutely been numerous bulls standing in front of me breathing steam onto those glasses (ones that usually answer to the name "Organic Chemistry"). But instead of taking them off to clean them with the risk of damaging those precious lenses, I simply hold my ground and wait for the bull to leave. Eventually the fog starts to clear and I begin on my path again. I am not sure how long the road is, but I know there will be so many great things to experience along the way and I look forward to growing even more along the way.

The student returns to her rose-colored glasses theme again and weaves in some more details which distract from her message. This is a good example of a student trying to get too creative with a personal statement. The bull "breathing steam" and waiting for the fog to clear are examples of phrases that are too creative for this kind of piece. There is a picture of a boy in Syria that most people have seen. This is the only story of a "patient" that the student wrote about. How am I supposed to know that she wants to be a physician based on this? With her story, maybe she wants to be a social worker? Maybe she should go work for a non-governmental organization?

Based on the above draft, I would tell this student to go back and look at her journey. I would tell her to think about what has shaped her desire to be a physician and what makes her stand out as an individual. She possibly could write about her struggles with depression as a way to stand out, just as a student wrote about his addiction, which likely earned him an interview. I need to see more experiences related to being a physician, so I know this is what she wants to do.

NL FINAL DRAFT

I haven't always known that I wanted to be a doctor. But my decision to become a physician is woven out of various influential threads of my life, such as my fascination with the human body, a desire to serve others, a natural ease with leadership, and my experience teaching. These are the threads of this story, which lead me now into the field of medicine.

> *Here we're greeted with another mission statement type opening.* **Telling me this type of information is usually just wasted characters because they** *know* *that you want to be a doctor, you just need to* **show** *them through your personal journey, not just by shouting it from the rooftops like this. Why does she want to be a doctor? A "fascination with the human body" and a "desire to serve others." This is the same as saying you like science and want to help people. You have to think bigger.*

My love of the human body was first expressed as an artist, studying dance in college. While pursuing my degree, it surprised me how enchanted I was with the scientific study of the body. My coursework in Anatomy, Physiology, and Kinesiology proved as engaging and intriguing as my work a dancer. After graduation, my goal was both to feed this excitement for the scientific study of the body and to serve others. These two desires interlaced beautifully in my practice as a nationally certified massage therapist. Through this vocation, I have continued to study how the body works, how it best functions, and the causes of imbalance and dysfunction. Additionally, this profession affords me the joy of helping clients feel less pain and stress, as well as the ability to craft a plan of care in partnership with each client. In these close relationships with clients over years of clinical practice, I have developed and honed interpersonal, team, and practical skills that will be invaluable as a physician, such as: taking health histories, asking keen questions, balancing compassionate care with efficiency, an understanding of referral relationships, knowledge of integrative healing modalities, and solid communication skills.

> *This paragraph gives us some useful information about the student. First, she is a nontraditional applicant, having worked as a massage therapist for a while. She writes about healing and helping her clients, and gives me a sense that she understands the relationship between a healer and a patient. She could have told a story of one particular client and how she helped him/her. It would have been a better* showing *paragraph if something like that were incorporated.*
> *See how this student sells her skills in the last sentence. This isn't needed. By* telling *me that she was a massage therapist, I already understand that she probably has a lot of these skills.* Show *me, through your story. Don't* tell *me by trying to sell your skills.*

I also weave my knowledge and excitement for human anatomy into the teaching curriculum of the Anatomy and Physiology section of 200-hour yoga teacher training programs. I have been asked regularly to train new teachers in this segment of various courses around the country. Over many years of teaching this material, I refined my ability to present complex concepts to an audience with widely varying backgrounds and comfort with scientific material. I deliver the topics in a relatable way. By weaving students lived experiences, yogic philosophies as well as concrete anatomy and physiology concepts together I keep the students engaged in the study. My prowess of presentation and my ability to keep the material fresh had my students and fellow teachers asking for a resource that brought all of my understanding together in one place. This led me to write and publish, the book, Enlightened Bodies: Physical and Subtle Human Anatomy.

This paragraph doesn't tell me anything more about the student and her desire to be on this path to medicine. Finding out she is an author does add to her personal story and helps her be unique, but we're still very far away from learning why she wants to be a doctor.

My ties to the yoga community are deep and personally satisfying, and have also developed me as a leader. After first attending one of the twice-yearly Solstice Yoga Festivals in 2008, I volunteered in the office and quickly rose through the ranks to become the event manager by 2011. As an integral member of the leadership team charged with marshaling the complex logistics needed to coordinate 2000 people in a remote area for 10 days, I coordinated the work of teams of volunteers, mediated conflicts, and organized resources to deliver on the intricate needs of the event. As a leader, I balanced giving both specific instructions as well as autonomy to my volunteers, in order for them to feel ownership of their elements of the event, all the while I maintained a high-level view of the vast overarching logistics.

This is a textbook example of an extracurricular description in a personal statement. The student is selling her skills as a leader with this example but not furthering her story of becoming a physician. This would actually work really well as an extracurricular description, but not in the personal statement.

I believe that we live the most meaningful, most powerful, and most purposeful life when we serve others. Service has been the constant thread woven into my career as a massage therapist, along with my relationships within my yoga community. In addition, I intend to continue weaving a dedication to service through my career as a physician and my life. I hope to serve in the National Health Service Corps and practice in underserved populations. I also intend to serve as a leader in the emerging relationship between conventional and complementary modes of care. I value being of service. Knowing that I can continue to serve others in my new career is exciting and highly motivating.

This is a good "here's what I plan to do with my future" type comment.

It is now clear that the tapestry I am creating of service, of caring, of leadership, of a fascination with human anatomy, and of teaching is taking shape as the story of a physician becoming. The time is right for me to study medicine. The time is also right within the field of medicine for someone with my skills, knowledge, and unconventional history. As healthcare becomes more integrated, I am perfectly positioned to help patients regain health through the panoply of traditional and complementary modalities of care. I am ready to challenge myself by deepening my knowledge of the body, illness and treatments, to continue and expand my wholehearted life of service, to lead and teach and work as part of a healthcare team, and to heal, diagnose and comfort people with the best approaches to health.

The student ties together her nontraditional path well by giving a pitch that someone with her background is needed in medicine. This helps her stand out, but it isn't really necessary because she has already mentioned enough about herself as a massage therapist and nontraditional student.

After reading this, I'm left wanting more information about her experience with patients and Western medicine. How am I supposed to know that she is going to like being inside the medical system enough to get through medical school and residency? That would be my main lingering question. I would invite her for an interview and make sure to focus my questioning around that.

This student is attending an allopathic medical school in the Midwest.

SC FINAL DRAFT

Born into a family of lawyers and engineers, I never considered a career in Medicine until I moved from my home country of Brazil to the United States when I was thirteen years old. I have always had a fascination for human physiology due to the numerous visits I paid to emergency rooms as a child for injuries sustained while playing. While still in high school, I discovered the opportunity to receive a certification as a nurse assistant and sought after it knowing it would place me in an experienced position as my college years neared. I credit this education as a catalyst for pursuing medicine. At the time, nursing seemed the obvious career choice. However, after observing in the hospital setting how nurses were often underappreciated and underpaid for the amount of work they are assigned to do, and even scolded by physicians who were angry they were awakened in the middle of the night to manage an emergent patient, I became disenchanted. This experience inspired me to switch career paths; I wanted to be a catalyst for change. I knew I could be a better director of collaborative care while still exhibiting kindness and respect to the members of the healthcare team despite the time of day.

Here we're given a well-told story of a nontraditional immigrant to the US. This automatically means this student is different and I want to learn more. There are a couple things mentioned that I would leave out. Writing about pay, even though it's from the nurse's angle, is something I would completely leave out of a personal statement. You don't want me to think you are going into this for money. There are many other things to do to make more money, and faster, than being a physician. I would also leave out the part about nurses being scolded by physicians. Are there angry physicians who yell? Sure. But when you put it in a personal statement, you're shining light on negativity—and it's better to stay positive in a personal statement. Right now it reads like her "seed" is that she wants to be a doctor because doctors yell at nurses.

At times I thought my ambitions of becoming a physician would never be realized. My undergraduate studies have been halted or severely curbed on multiple occasions due to high-risk pregnancies and caring for my husband who sustained a traumatic brain injury, as he is currently in the final stages of recovery. However, I do not believe in quitting, even if it is the easier, and more practical choice. I took a stand and made a change within myself. I first took care of my life as I learned to balance my health and personal needs so that I could have the energy and positive attitude needed to care for those I loved. My journey to losing more than eighty pounds and overcoming clinical depression with the use of Beachbody fitness programs evolved into an even bigger sense of purpose, as I was inspired to help others become healthier through participation in fitness challenge groups. Halfway through my weight loss, I began coaching as a means to keep the accountability I strived to have with my own health, and as well as teaching those who are ready for a lifestyle change. Caring for my family and inspiring others to transform and seeing lives improved is rewarding, yet not completely fulfilling because I lack the skills necessary in managing their overall plan of medical care.

> *Here we're presented with plenty of information. The first is that the student has had a lot of setbacks. This may be reflected in her transcript. It may have taken her a long time to finish undergrad based on this info. She may have bad grades because of these experiences.*
> *It's a good red flag statement.*
> *She also works in what she did to overcome some of these obstacles, and she even incorporates the fact that she was unable to fulfill the needs of her fitness clients, motivating her to continue on this journey.*

I need to be a physician so I can be on the forefront of the fight against obesity and its health-related complications. Preventive medicine is of utmost importance to me, and not only so, looking at the patient as a whole human being and a set of interconnected systems, rather than a compilation of symptoms. The top three killers in our country are diseases related to poor diet choices. I can no longer sit idly on the sidelines as I had for several years, working in healthcare yet not being an example of health and personal accountability. As I worked for Intermountain Healthcare, I found that although the healthcare system went to great lengths to provide the patients with high quality and low-cost care, as highlighted by President Barack Obama, the night shift staff had limited choices on healthy food options and did not, until recently, provide incentives to help their employees live more active lifestyles. I hope my passion may also inspire my future physician colleagues by demonstrating that as they share their personal stories of how they have learned to maintain a consistent and balanced active life with the high demands of being a physician, their patients will feel an exponentially more powerful effect than simply being encouraged with hollow words. My goal is that my story and vision for healing will show them that healing begins with improving their own health first. I believe the process for changing ourselves will allow us to be more empathetic toward our patients but also inspire our patients to heed our recommendations. My hope is that this change in perspective will result in less time treating illness and rather preventing illness altogether.

After reading this paragraph, I want to stand up and cheer for this student. I feel pumped. I feel like we're going into battle against poor lifestyle choices. This is a great ending that shows what this student hopes to do in the future. I would have liked to see an example of her getting some experience, proving to me that being a physician is what she wants. I want to see that moment of reflection that says, "Yes, I have seen what doctors can do, and this is what I want."
This student was accepted to an osteopathic medical school in the South.

SR FINAL DRAFT

Trained as a graphic designer with limited medical knowledge, my life dramatically shifted when my mother suffered a massive heart attack that required emergency bypass heart surgery in 2012. Following the surgery, she was in a coma, faced a grueling recovery, and suffered many complications, including amputation of both feet, end-stage congestive heart failure, and several bouts of septic shock before passing away 10 months later. Over the course of her weakening state, I took on the role of caregiver and point person for my family. I spoke with doctors, attended appointments, relayed sensitive information, provided wound care, and organized her treatment plans at home. This role was a natural fit—I found a sense of purpose in managing her care and a developing interest in osteopathic medicine as I gained more exposure to the medical field. I vividly remember a conversation I shared with my mother in which she asked how much longer I thought she would live. I told her never to give up, that her life was not over, that she survived her heart attack for a reason, and that it did not matter what brought her to this point. She was alive and given a second chance to be the person she always sought to be. At the time, I was unaware that I would be following that same advice in my own pursuits of becoming an osteopathic physician.

This is the "seed." The student tells *us about being a nontraditional student as a graphic designer and about her mother suffering from a heart attack and all of the complications that arose after that. It could have been made a little more memorable, or stronger, with more* showing *statements. As an example, she could have written, "Sitting at the bedside, watching the nurses and doctors move about the room as my mother lie there motionless, in a coma, my life shifted dramatically." Just a small change in how the story is told alters it from* telling *to* showing. *This student applied to DO schools and in my mind, forced in the use of "osteopathic" into this paragraph. I don't think it's needed here.*

As weeks in the hospital turned to months, I found myself captivated by this dynamic environment. I soaked in as much information as I could and enjoyed learning the various medical landscapes. Experiencing the entire continuum of care first hand, I learned how a hospital works, learning about the emergency department, intensive care unit, skilled nursing facility, physical and occupational therapy, home healthcare, and a routine clinic appointment. Much of my mother's rehabilitation was spent at skilled nursing facilities in Pittsburgh, Pennsylvania. This was my first direct exposure to urban healthcare and I began to see some of the biopsychosocial challenges faced within this environment: poor diet, lack of support, abuse, and socioeconomic difficulties. Through this process, I spent time contemplating the genesis of how conditions escalated. It became apparent that illness is not simply a state of diseased tissue; it is the result of a culmination of many factors. I soon discovered that my contemplations were directly in line with the philosophy behind osteopathic medicine, in which to fully treat a patient, we must examine them in a holistic manner.

We're given more backstory and reference to the exposure that the student had while caring for her mother. Writing about how she learned how a hospital works and the purpose of each of the departments seems like a waste of space that could have been better utilized on other details. Remember, knowing how a hospital works or knowing about a physician's role, does not mean you should be a doctor.
At the end of this paragraph, she starts to bring in more information about her motivations. Here, the use of osteopathic medicine seems appropriate because she is drawing lines directly to some of what the osteopathic world markets itself as entailing.

After my mother's death, I was filled with an overwhelming urge to take action. I spent time volunteering, researching disease prevention and patient experience. I knew that my story was not unique on a macroscopic level; society must be aware of the detrimental effects of lifestyle choices. I quickly learned that these issues were complicated, that lifestyle is sometimes not a choice, but can be dictated by cultural beliefs and socioeconomic status. I needed to fully invest myself in medicine to be on the forefront of action, so I enrolled in a post-baccalaureate premed program at University where I received a second Bachelor's in Health Sciences with a 3.85 GPA. In addition to the solid foundation I have gained in the premedical sciences, I have had more exposure to urban health in the communities of Pittsburgh, taken courses in urban, community, and cultural health, as well as biomedical ethics. I continually strive to better understand all walks of life and motivations that may influence lifestyle and medical decisions to better myself as a future DO.

> **Telling *vs.* showing.** *If you don't take anything else away from this book, take that away. This paragraph is all* telling. *"I spent time." "I quickly learned." "I needed to fully invest." Not only is this* telling *me what the student was doing, it goes into a list of next steps. I don't need to see the timeline and I definitely don't need to see where the student went to school and what her GPA was. The last few sentences could have been told as a little story about volunteering in the community, getting the exposure that she is* telling *me about. It would have been more memorable that way. The reference to DO in the last sentence still feels forced to me. Understanding all walks of life is great for all physicians, not just DOs.*

These experiences have directly impacted my trajectory in life to pursue a career as an osteopathic physician with a mission to educate and empower patients on disease prevention. What happened to my mother could have been prevented through lifestyle modifications and proper education earlier in life. Today, many Americans are unaware that cardiac symptoms may manifest differently in women. I have become an advocate to my community and social circles, promoting the "silent symptoms" of heart disease in women; however, more work must be done. As an osteopathic medical student, I will gain the tools necessary to succeed in a field that aligns with my passion for preventative and lifestyle medicine in hopes of breaking the cycle and inspiring change in my community.

This last paragraph is an effective ending that discusses what the student hopes to achieve as a medical student and physician. The osteopathic references here are still forced and aren't needed. If you are mentioning something very specific that ties into osteopathic medicine, do so. For example, earlier, she referred to disease as a culmination of many factors and then wrote about osteopathic medicine. While allopathic physicians also consider other factors, this is a good tie-in to osteopathic medicine because that is the marketing that they use. The other references are just about being a doctor in general, and osteopathic medicine doesn't need to be forced into this.
This student is attending an osteopathic medical school in the Midwest.

VY FINAL DRAFT

Having to decide on a future career at a young age was a difficult choice for me to make. There was an entire world of careers, each different and unique, but which path was meant for me? This confusion made me feel as if I was stuck in a jungle and the only way out was that I had to explore my interests to open a path to my future. My interest in medicine first piqued when I took my first anatomy and physiology class in high school. I was amazed by the complexity of the human body and how all of the systems in the body functioned together to keep the body alive. My desire to continue learning about the human body combined with my experiences as an EMT, volunteering and shadowing an osteopathic physician have all provided for me a path out of the jungle and into the world of medicine.

This opening was highlighted earlier in the book under what to avoid. The first thing is the jungle theme. It needs to go. I think you can see by now that themes just don't belong in a personal statement.
The second thing is the use of very general statements. Yes, deciding on a career is difficult, for everyone. Yes, there are a lot of unique careers. Yes, you need to explore your interests to figure out the best path forward. Each of these is a very general statement that doesn't need to be there. What was the "seed?" Anatomy and physiology and being an EMT. That's the biggest takeaway from this paragraph.

The flashing lights and loud sirens of the ambulances in my town always left me intrigued and curious to know how ordinary people were saving lives at a high speed. My curiosity drew me to volunteer as a certified EMT at my hometown Rescue Squad. One day, while on call, an elderly patient had slipped and fallen on the ground. Treating for a spinal injury, the other EMTs and I, worked together to attach a cervical collar and backboard the patient onto a stretcher. Working as a unit, we delegated roles: I was in charge of stabilizing the head, two other EMTs were in charge of log-rolling the patient, and the fourth had to slide the backboard under. To prevent any miscalculated actions that could prove detrimental to the patient, I told my team to "log roll on three," and proceeded to count to three. In such an experience, I learned that by coordinating our actions, we can move towards treating the patient more efficiently and effectively. The skills I gained as an EMT to function in a team successfully will be an asset for my future colleagues and patients.

This is a decent paragraph. It could have been the start of the personal statement. It would have been made stronger with a little more about the experience with the patient, and not just focusing on the communication and teamwork skills she gained as an EMT. The takeaway is centered around the skills of teamwork and not around being a physician or the impact she had on the patient.

Since I was nine years old, I have been attending a religious summer camp every year. As an EMT, I was qualified to care for the health of the campers. My knowledge from EMT training proved useful when I encountered a camper who was having trouble breathing. He was sitting on his bed, hunched forward and wheezing. My EMT training immediately directed me to treat him as an anaphylactic patient. I quickly administered him an EpiPen, and then sat with him to monitor his vitals. After he normalized, he gave me a hug and said "thank you, you saved my life." It was at this moment that I felt an overwhelming sense of gratification and happiness. This camp was a second home for me, and for me to be able to use my knowledge to save those that I considered family was heartwarming and reassuring of the path I was following. Treating the child made me eager to expand my knowledge of medicine and determine to become a physician so that I could provide care to a broader community. I was slowly making my way out of the jungle.

This is better. The takeaway was about the patient and the emotions surrounding caring for the camper. The jungle reference could be deleted.

Shadowing Dr. Smith, an osteopathic cardiologist, solidified my decision to pursue a career in medicine. In one instance, Dr. Smith was called to the ER to consult a patient who had fainted and was reported to have an irregular heartbeat. The patient was unaware of her heart condition and instead believed that she was dehydrated. She became anxious of her future upon learning of her heart condition; however, Dr. Smith took her hand and told her that there was nothing to worry about. He used simple vocabulary to show how her heart was beating, and reassured her that her symptoms were common and treatable. The way he delivered hope and reassurance to his patient reminded me of the reason why I started a Global Medical Brigades chapter at my school. I noticed my peers changing their career paths and navigating through their own jungles. In understanding their struggles, I provided them an opportunity where they could volunteer abroad in medical clinics and solidify their own decision to pursue medicine. My genuine compassion for others will enable me to be a successful physician.

This paragraph started very well, but then took a very sharp turn with the comparison to Global Medical Brigades (GMB). I don't know what the student was trying to accomplish here, other than making sure that I knew that she started a GMB chapter. In a previous personal statement, I mentioned how the student showed me she was compassionate through the use of her words. This is the exact opposite. The student is telling me that she is compassionate. It comes off much more effectively with the former approach.

Escaping the jungle helped me find my way to medicine. My experiences have guided me in my path to pursue medicine. Being able to use the knowledge of the human body to impact people's lives would be the best way to give back to a world I owe so much to. Though the journey is long, I believe that I possess the curiosity, dedication and interpersonal skills needed to continue my path towards medicine.

> *What does this student hope to accomplish? Where is her big vision for the future? The last sentence is a great example of a student describing skills she thinks I want to see. "Curiosity, dedication, and interpersonal skills" are good skills to have, but definitely aren't unique to this student and aren't unique to being a physician. The student was invited for an interview at an osteopathic medical school in the South.*

SH FINAL DRAFT

I followed the surgeon into the room and saw a young woman, anxious about the lump she had found in her breast. My mind brought me back to when my mom, in her late 30s, sat us down and told us she was dying from breast cancer. Given the emotional magnitude of the patient's situation, I was surprised when she seemed to relax as the doctor explained the procedure. The doctor helped ease the patient's fear by teaching her about the procedure with a calm demeanor and straightforward language. This surgeon, who was also my stepmother, showed me that while doctors cannot save every life, they can have a profound impact by helping to comfort and educate their patients.

This student starts her personal statement with an affecting story of shadowing and the interesting twist that the surgeon she was with was her stepmother. The student shows us one of her initial exposures to medicine, her mother's breast cancer.

Inspired by my two moms, I started college premed. I fell in love with chemistry and started tutoring with the TRiO program, a program that targets veterans, minorities, and first-generation students. I was struck by the resilience and motivation of my students, and captivated by the feeling of making an impact. My newfound passion for teaching drove me to put my premed aspirations to the side and focus on building a career in higher education.

We learn that the student found a passion for teaching and stopped being premed. This sets the statement up for an insightful story about reflection later.

I discovered a master's program where I could apply my crystallography research to a new field while teaching. The program seemed idyllic; it challenged me academically and allowed me to teach. However, I quickly found that I missed working with underserved populations. I began volunteering as a domestic violence emergency responder. Through this, my passion for serving people struggling with mental illness and oppression grew.

> *The student jumps right into an experience in which she was able to reflect and realize that she enjoyed working with those with mental illnesses. See how she didn't just say she found a passion for serving people? She specifically mentioned people struggling with mental illness.*

As a teacher, I continued to encounter mental illness. One afternoon, I opened an email with a benign title: "HW 4 makeup". "I spent the morning contemplating suicide," the student had written. I quickly wrote back, mentioning resources, asking questions, and offering support. The student and I continued to talk; she found support and reported improvement throughout the semester. In the aftermath of this event, I wanted to do more for students like her. I trained in mental health intervention and advocacy, but remained frustrated by my limitations. I began to think that if I were a physician, I could more directly help my students.

> *This story brings the student full circle to the realization that medicine and being a physician was where she needed to be. This is reflection. This is a great takeaway.*

Around this time, my colleague often spoke passionately about how his son's doctors changed the lives of his family. Sam, his son, has congenital hydrocephalus and has had six brain surgeries in five years. One weekend, I took Sam rock climbing. He whooped when he reached the peak of the wall and came down gasping. "I did it! I got to the top!" In that moment, I realized that Sam's doctors had given him a life full of potential. My colleague connected me with Sam's surgeon, and two weeks later I crowded into a busy operating room. That day, after 3 hours of surgery,

6-month-old Samantha woke up with a new life ahead of her. I watched her sit up and I thought, "This is what I need to do." I was thrilled by the opportunity to solve health problems and create a lasting impact on a child's life.

> *The student cleverly works in a story of shadowing and being around patients. Her takeaway shows that she knows she is on the right path.*

My motivation was reaffirmed when I shadowed internal medicine in downtown Seattle. During rounds, we met a patient admitted for alcohol withdrawal. The doctor knelt down next to the patient and said, "You are my favorite type of patient, because you still have the chance to be healthy. If you stop drinking now, you can still have a full life." I could hear the sincerity in the doctor's voice; and evidently the patient could too, because she asked how she could move forward. The patient's trust allowed the doctor to be a strong advocate for change. I realized as a physician, I could merge my passion for teaching with my desire to heal and treat.

> *Here we see another story from the student's journey. This is an excellent example of an extracurricular which belongs in the personal statement. It isn't **telling** us about the extracurricular. It's **showing** us why the extracurricular was such an impactful part of her story.*

While I enjoyed shadowing, I was still not sure that I would like working with the sick and dying, so I began volunteering with hospice patients. The first day I came into Jane's room, she motioned for me to sit down on a hard plastic chair. We began chatting, and within an hour, she told me about how her husband had died, followed by her son, then followed the murder of her daughter. I was astounded. After she told me, she looked out the window and said, "You don't think about it too much. Only when the weather is cloudy." That day, Jane exemplified what I have seen in many hospice patients. They are vulnerable, candid, and often resilient. They leave me wanting to do everything I can to ease their burdens.

> *The student weaves in another story about working directly with patients, reaffirming her passions.*

Volunteering with hospice patients helped me understand that working with sick and dying people is a uniquely challenging and fulfilling task. Their vulnerability allows doctors to form intimate relationships that carry tremendous responsibility. As a premed in college, I was uncertain whether I could carry this responsibility. Now, I have realized I am driven to serve people to my highest potential. I will be satisfied with nothing less than having the full responsibility of their care, so that I can do everything in my power to improve their lives. As a doctor, I will heal, educate, and advocate for patients like my mother, Sam, and Jane.

The student closes the personal statement with a great statement of reflection, describing being uncertain of her initial path. She's able to show the Admissions Committee that her journey has done nothing but reaffirm her passion for medicine and that she is ready for the next step. This student has received multiple acceptances to allopathic medical schools.

IC FINAL DRAFT

On June 13, 2004, I woke up in the middle of the night to two strangers telling me to get up and get dressed. My mother then came to my room with tears in her eyes. It did not feel like it then, but this was my second chance at life. The strangers were employees of a drug rehabilitation program sent to take me for treatment. A year later, I graduated and celebrated my first year of sobriety. Through this challenging experience, I realized the sacrifices my mother had made. After my parents separated, she worked long hours at a hair salon in order to support the two of us. As an immigrant from a farming town in Hong Kong, she never had the opportunity to make it past middle school. But eventually she saved enough to purchase a home - the same home she sold 12 years later to afford my rehabilitation program. She took a gamble in the hopes that she could give me an opportunity to live the life she envisioned when she immigrated to America. Today I feel an immense sense of responsibility to do the best I can. This sense of responsibility has culminated into my drive to become a physician who can treat disease and thereby positively influence the lives others.

This student immediately hits me in the face with a potential red flag: drug addiction. Notice how she didn't dwell on it though.
She does a great job of mentioning it and moving on to tell me more about her story as the daughter of an immigrant. She tells me a great story of the sacrifice her mother made and gives me a glimpse at her drive and motivation. This is a very good opening.

Attending this rehabilitation program changed the trajectory of my life. After graduating, I immediately enrolled myself in community college and applied for my first job. I decided to pursue a degree in psychology to help others dealing with addiction. I transferred to State University where I graduated with my bachelors degree in psychology. Although I wanted to further my education, it was not financially feasible at that time. I postponed my dreams of becoming a mental health provider to work full-time as an office manager in a chiropractic office and financially support my mother. After saving money for a couple of years, I started a masters program in marriage and family therapy at State University while continuing to work full-time. I became the first person in my family to receive a graduate degree.

We start to get into a timeline of the student's journey, which isn't needed. There are some very interesting parts here that could have stood alone, outside of the timeline format. The student delaying more schooling to support her mother shows her dedication to her family and potential dedication to her future patients. See how she didn't say, "I'm dedicated to patients," but it still reads that way. This is the difference between showing and telling.

Upon completion of my graduate degree, I began an internship in mental health at State Hospital (SH). Here, I became more interested in providing comprehensive healthcare that extended beyond mental health as I participated in rounds with pediatricians. It was gratifying to be part of a team that included physicians, nurses, nutritionists, speech therapists, and case managers. At SH, my passion for medicine was reaffirmed when I witnessed physicians provide treatments to their patients. This resonated with me because as a physician, I would be able to utilize my medical knowledge to critically think about the disease processes and offer appropriate treatments. I was also further inspired to enter medicine when I observed care that centered on building relationships with patients in order to earn their trust and achieve better medical outcomes.

> *Here is more timeline information about an experience that "reaffirmed" the student's desire to enter medicine. I love the use of this word. This could have been made much stronger by showing being part of the team, instead of just the telling that the student does here.*

I learned more about the medical profession while serving as a clinical research coordinator with the County Department of Health in Georgia. In this role, I work closely with infectious disease specialists at the State University. My responsibilities include screening patients with HIV, taking medical histories, and communicating with patients regularly. I have gained an appreciation for this disease that extends beyond what I had learned in my biology textbooks. Every day, I have the privilege of getting a glimpse into the lives of patients who struggle with adherence to drug cocktails or viral load suppression. It has been incredible to see how a strong physician-patient relationship results in better adherence to medications and more regular follow up. Also, my desire to learn medicine increased as I witnessed the complex and multidisciplinary nature of HIV management.

> *The student continues with another extracurricular that shows her that this is the journey for her. Just like in the previous paragraph, this could have been made much stronger through the use of showing statements. For example, with the sentence, "I have the privilege of getting a glimpse into the lives of patients who struggle with adherence to drug cocktails or viral load suppression," the student could have told us a story about interacting with one of these patients. It could have been almost as short and would have been a much more powerful way to engage my senses as the reader.*

I believe my experiences as a mental health professional would help me better connect with patients as a future physician. During my time as a volunteer therapist for County Family Service and the County Health Care Agency, I worked to build relationships with the patients I served by empathetically listening to them and involving them in care decisions. I had the opportunity to work with patients from many different cultures and learned to be sensitive towards beliefs about mental health. These lessons can be transferred into the medical profession, where I would also work with diverse populations. I understand that patients may have anxiety, worry, or depression surrounding their illness. I look forward to drawing on my background in mental health to address patients' psychological wellbeing while also treating their ailments.

This is another example of a great experience that could be made into a much more impactful paragraph through the use of showing and not telling. The student uses a very good example of a telling statement: "I worked to build relationships with the patients I served by empathetically listening to them and involving them in care decisions." With just a few changes to how this is written, it would have showed me that she was empathetic, instead of her telling me. What if she had said: "Jane sat in front of me, just as she did every month. I couldn't stop picturing what her life was like as she explained some of her difficulties getting to the doctor's office. With that knowledge, we worked together to make sure that moving forward, we did everything possible to get her the care she needed." This is longer, but it shows me that the student is engaged, and being empathetic, instead of just her telling me that she is.

My journey has had quite a bit of twists and turns as I went from a recovering addict to a mental health therapist to a successful premedical student. I believe my unique personal and professional experiences will help me contribute a different perspective to patient care. Every event in my life from my own struggle with substance abuse to my work in mental health and my service in the HIV infected population has reinvigorated my desire to become a physician. I look forward to entering this profession and serving vulnerable communities as a compassionate medical doctor who got a second chance.

The student does a great job of wrapping up and telling me what she hopes to accomplish once she becomes a physician. She could have left out some of the comments about being a successful premed student and her perspective on how her background will help her be a physician, but overall, this essay does what it needs to do. It lets me know why she is on this journey and what has continued to reaffirm for her that she is on the right path. I think this could have been improved with some small tweaks, but overall it achieved its goal: it got her an interview. This student has had multiple interviews and is currently holding an acceptance to a Midwest allopathic medical school.

CK FINAL DRAFT

Desperate for medical attention, but afraid of going to the emergency room for fear of deportation, the migrant farm worker fought back tears as he held his severely infected hand. Hoping to save his hand and livelihood, he sat next to me in the waiting area of La Clinica, a free migrant clinic. I was reading to the children of patients when he returned from being seen by the volunteer doctors; the relief across his face embodied the significant difference a caring physician could make. That moment pushed me to reflect on my adoption and the opportunities it afforded me.

> *This is an intriguing opening about the student volunteering at a clinic. There are some good* **showing** *statements which make me picture what is going on. I'm interested in the transition to being adopted and wonder where the student is taking me.*

My biological father and mother, with me in utero, emigrated from El Salvador, hoping to find jobs to pay for the transit of their children. My father didn't survive the harrowing journey and my mother couldn't complete their dream alone. Realizing this, she selflessly gave me up for adoption before returning to her children in El Salvador. Altruistically, my parents adopted me at a time when they had two children and two careers filling their lives. These events are what guided me towards serving the underprivileged as I grew up.

> *This student* **shows** *me his past and how it has shaped him and driven him to where he is today and who he wants to be in the future.*

While volunteering at a homeless shelter, I had the privilege of working with clients from diverse social, ethnic, and economic backgrounds. Some were newly homeless while others had accepted homelessness as their lifestyle. The patient population included those who were mentally ill, substance abusers, newly released prisoners, veterans, the physically disabled, and "working girls"—my experiences at the shelter were as diverse as the clients we assisted. I gave a series of lectures on a variety of health related topics such as sun protection, dehydration, and hypertension. At first, attendance was discouragingly low, but picked up dramatically beginning with my talk on sex safety. It was during the discussion sessions following the educational lectures that I became privy to lifestyles, beliefs, and perspectives that I had never considered. For instance, many of the "working girls" fell into the cycle of homelessness after engaging in "survival sex", a means of fleeing from physically or sexually abusive home situations. This experience has broadened my awareness and deepened my understanding of the obstacles and challenges faced by those who are marginalized by society. It has strengthened my resolve to become a physician for all people, regardless of their culture, lifestyle, beliefs, and socioeconomic status.

This student falls into the common trap of trying to tie everything to being a physician. How does having your awareness broadened and understanding deepened about the obstacles and challenges faced by those who are marginalized make you want to be a physician? Why not be a social worker to help those people? You could become a politician or work at a non-profit to drive change for these people.
If you are going to tie something to furthering your desire to be a physician, make sure that it clearly makes sense why.

I've had the privilege of shadowing a number of talented physicians. There is one in particular, Dr. Smith, whose interactions with patients so impressed me that they significantly reinforced my decision to study medicine. As an experienced, 75-year-old neurologist, he taught me a lot about neurology during the month that I shadowed him. The thing that captivated me most, though, was the way in which he interacted and connected with patients and their loved ones. Dr. Smith regularly has to give diagnoses with bleak prognoses, such as Parkinson's and Alzheimer's disease. These disorders are incurable and progressively degenerative, facts Dr. Smith has to explain without causing distress. In the face of what appears to be a no-win situation, Dr. Smith adeptly weaves his explanation into a passionate plan of action—with a powerful, hopeful, and upbeat tone, he elaborates on what to expect, and exactly how they'll all face it together. Their belief in Dr. Smith's words grow as he goes on to assure his patient that, with the supportive team comprised of physician, patient, and loved ones, he or she will move forward from these circumstances, make the most of what they have, and lead a fulfilling life. By the end of the appointment, the patient's expression is one of gratitude and resilience instead of fear and sadness. I know from my background in the behavioral sciences that medical outcomes are improved when patients feel connected to their medical providers; I'm confident that I can make this connection with patients and am excited about this critically important aspect of medicine.

In this paragraph, the student discusses a shadowing experience but doesn't help the reader connect with the patient care aspect. Instead, the student focuses on the physician. It is good, but it could have been much better if he had told the story of a patient and their family getting a devastating diagnosis and how he wants to help in those situations.

My interest in the physical and biological sciences, strong background in behavioral sciences, and my desire to have the greatest impact in helping people lead me to pursue a career in medicine. I believe that I possess the intellectual ability, empathy, and passion for helping people to be a great physician.

This first sentence could be summed up as, "I like science and want to help people, so I want to be a physician." Just because you possess the smarts, empathy, and passion to be a physician, doesn't mean you should be one. This statement is just the student making sure that the reader checks off those boxes on the "Traits Applicant Has" checklist. This isn't needed. Finish with how you hope to have an impact on the world, your patients, and your community.

The student has had very interesting experiences, but he could have conveyed them more effectively in this personal statement. This is a good example of a personal statement that would require a look at the secondary essays. I'd need to know more about this student to see if I'd want to interview him.

This student is a current medical student at an osteopathic medical school in the South.

CLOSING

The hardest part about writing this book was being careful not to tell you *what* to put in your personal statement, but rather *how* to tell your story. I know that after reading this book and following the advice given, as well as reading the example personal statements and feedback, that you will be able to craft a great personal statement which *shows* the Admissions Committee *who* you are and *why* they need to invite you for an interview.

If you're reading this early on in your journey, start journaling. After every experience, make a note of why that event was so impactful for you. Remember, it's not just the *what*, but the *why* that truly matters.

Start your first draft several months out from when you plan on applying to medical school (or postbac). The personal statement is not something you want to rush through. After each draft, try to go back to it with fresh eyes and look at it from the reader's perspective. Does it tell you *why* you are doing this? If it does, great. If it doesn't, don't be afraid to start fresh.

Most of all, please remember that your journey is unique. Don't try to force things into your personal statement to stand out; it doesn't work. Take the reader on a voyage through your experiences and convey why they are important enough to write about in your essay. Show them why this is so important to you and what you hope to accomplish after getting your medical degree.

Reflect on your past experiences and dream big about your goals. Write your best story and secure your interview! (Then go check out *The Premed Playbook: Guide to the Medical School Interview*.)

ABOUT THE AUTHOR

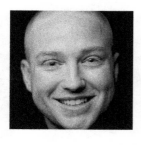 Dr. Ryan Gray is a former United States Air Force Flight Surgeon who found a passion for helping premed students on their journey to medical school. Best known for his podcasts, which have been downloaded over 2,000,000 times, Dr. Gray has interviewed numerous Admissions Committee members and deans of admissions for medical schools.

Through *The Premed Years* podcast and the Medical School Headquarters sites, Dr. Gray has helped thousands of students gain the confidence they require to successfully navigate the premed path.

Dr. Gray lives outside of Boulder, CO with his wife Allison, who is a Neurologist, and their daughter Hannah. Dr. Gray is also a Clinical Instructor at the University of Colorado School of Medicine.

Check out all of Dr. Gray's books at premedplaybook.com.

If you'd like Dr. Gray to speak to your premed club or at your conference, send an email to team@medicalschoolhq.net.

RESOURCES

WEBSITES

Medical School Headquarters: For the best information to help premeds on the path to medical school - https://medicalschoolhq.net.

PODCASTS

There are currently six podcasts on the Meded Media Network: *The Premed Years, OldPreMeds Podcast, The MCAT Podcast, Specialty Stories, Ask Dr. Gray: Premed Q&A, and The Shortcoat Podcast* – http://www.mededmedia.com.

PODCAST EPISODES ABOUT THE MEDICAL SCHOOL PERSONAL STATEMENT

The Premed Years

Session 38: How to Write Personal Statements with Dr. Vineet Arora (https://medicalschoolhq.net/38)

Session 88: Writing Personal Statements for Medical School (https://medicalschoolhq.net/88)

Session 127: The Medical School Application Personal Statement (https://medicalschoolhq.net/127)

Session 161: 5 Biggest Medical School Personal Statement Mistakes (https://medicalschoolhq.net/161)

OldPreMeds Podcast

AAMC AND AACOMAS RESOURCES

Medical School Admissions Requirements – https://medicalschoolhq.net/msar
College Information Book – https://medicalschoolhq.net/cib

PERSONAL STATEMENT EDITING

https://medicalschoolhq.net/personal-statement-editing/
Want to work directly with the Medical School Headquarters to help craft your perfect personal statement? Check out the many different services available by visiting the link above or by finding the Services menu on medicalschoolhq.net.

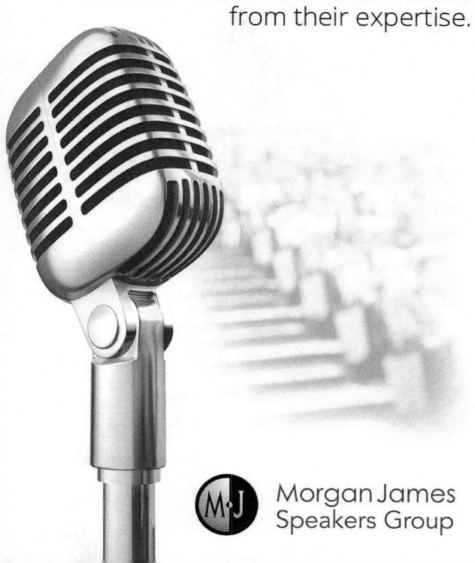

CPSIA information can be obtained
at www.ICGtesting.com
Printed in the USA
JSHW021436250921
19013JS00001B/20

9 781683 508533